Brain Robber and New Treatments for Alzheimer's Disease

Jane George

ATLANTIC
PUBLISHERS & DISTRIBUTORS (P) LTD

Published by
ATLANTIC
PUBLISHERS & DISTRIBUTORS (P) LTD
7/22, Ansari Road, Darya Ganj, New Delhi-110002
Phones : +91-11-40775252, 23273880, 23275880, 23280451
Fax : +91-11-23285873
Web : www.atlanticbooks.com
E-mail : orders@atlanticbooks.com

Branch Office
5, Nallathambi Street, Wallajah Road, Chennai-600002
Phones : +91-44-64611085, 32413319
E-mail : chennai@atlanticbooks.com

Printed in India at Nice Printing Press, A-33/3A, Site-IV, Industrial Area, Sahibabad, Ghaziabad, U.P.

Preface

The book deals with Alzheimer's disease (AD), a devastating progressive neurodegenerative brain disease that gradually destroys cognitive abilities including attention, concentration, language, thinking, abstraction, reasoning, memory, emotions, personality and behavior. Current research carried out at National Institute to Health (NIH) in USA and National Health Services (NHS) in Great Britain contribute wealth of informations as to the etiology of AD. Amyloid and Biomarkers are discussed. Clinical manifestation, different stages of AD, and Neuropsychological testing are laid out. Dysfunctions in detail of the Lobes of the brain and the neurotransmitters; and various forms of treatments are considered.

Future Drug treatment like PBT2, NeuroAD, and alternative treatments like Ayurveda, Homeopathy, herbal, cognitive retraining and other types of treatments are explored. Neuroimaging and latest Bioluminescence imaging that noninvasively monitor disease progression are explained. Various techniques to stimulate all the senses are suggested in order to maintain Cognitive abilities of Alzheimer's. There are chapters on various forms of pollution that affect the brain adversely. Caregiving, Social respite homes, Assisted Living and so forth are reviewed that will be beneficial and secure for the elderly. The very high personal cost, and societal cost are scrutinized. Preventive measures are suggested. Finally, Cognitive Stimulation Therapy that addresses all the symptoms of Alzheimer's, Habilitation and Rehabilitation therapeutic modalities are presented. The book will be of immense value to those who work with AD, physicians, professors, nurses, social workers, graduate students, and allied health professionals and those who take care of AD patients at home. Content of the book will be of help to the family members of the Alzheimer's patient.

Jane George

Contents

Preface .... *iii*

1. Brain Robber, New Treatments for Alzheimer's 1
2. Historical Background, Conceptual Perspective and Risk Factors 8
3. Pollution 49
4. Stages of Progression of Alzheimer's and Techniques for Evaluations 60
5. Lobes of the Brain and Their Functions 73
6. Neuropsychological Assessment 98
7. Current Treatment for Alzheimer's 133
8. Caregiving 202
9. Prevention 230
10. Cognitive Stimulation Therapy/Habilitation for Mild to Moderate Alzheimer's 246

1

Brain Robber, New Treatments for Alzheimer's

PREVALENCE OF ALZHEIMER'S IN INDIA

Alzheimer's disease (AD) is defined by Neuroscientists as an irreversible, progressive neurodegenerative brain disease that slowly destroys cognitive abilities including attention, concentration, language, thinking, abstraction, reasoning, speech, memory, emotions, personality and behavior. AD destroys billions of neurons in the brain incapacitating an individual to be successful in social and occupational functioning. AD attacks the brain's neurons which are vital in producing the brain chemical or neurotransmitter called acetylcholine, associated with memory and learning. Two types of abnormal lesions clog the brains of Alzheimer's: Beta-amyloid plaques and neurofibrillary tangles.

Prevalence

Alzheimer's disease affects currently around 5.43 million Americans of all ages. This includes 5.2 million people who are 65 years of age and older. 13 per cent of 65 year-olds have AD. It is reported that half of the people of 85 years of age and older have AD. By the middle of the century, 14 million Americans who are over 80 years of age will suffer from Alzheimer's. It is the fourth leading cause of death among elderly in USA (Perry 1995); and as reported by 2012 Alzheimer's Disease Facts and Figures.

G8 summit in London 2013 reported the statistics of Dementia across the globe as follows: 44 million globally have dementia. 135 million will have the disease in 2050. By 2050 71 per cent will be poor and middle income; 600bn dollars will be the global cost of Dementia. There are 3.7 million Indians with Dementia. This number is expected to double by 2030 and the cost will increase by three times.

The death registered in USA due to AD is more than 50,000 per year. AD is the most common cause of dementia in USA and it accounts for 50-70 per cent of the cases.

Alzheimer's news 2-13-2013: In his first state of the Union address of his second term, President Barak Obama of USA, spoke of "the need for investments in science and innovation", with a specific reference to Alzheimer's disease. He assigned several millions for research and several millions to spend every year to conduct research on Alzheimer's disease. In addition, 2014 budget, funds the National Institutes of Health's Brain Research through the Advancing Innovative Neurotechnologies (BRAIN) Initiative.

Prime Minister of UK David Cameron's dementia challenge: He has committed to more than doubling government spending, from £26.6 million in 2009-10, to an estimated £66.3 million in 2014-15.

The Obama administration is planning a decade long scientific effort to examine the workings of the human brain. Neuroscientists will be studying brain's billion neurons to understand the many facets of the brain.

Prior to scientific methods to diagnose Alzheimer's disease the diagnosis was made on the basis of Autopsy. McKhann (1984) reported that 20 per cent or more people clinically diagnosed with Alzheimer's are found at Autopsy did not have Alzheimer's disease at all.

In another Post-mortem study three out of 12 Alzheimer's patients actually died from a Spongy form Encephalopathy (Teixeira 1995).

In a recent report on Alzheimer's disease by World Health organization, it is estimated that there are 35.6 million people living with dementia worldwide in 2010, increasing to 65.7

million by 2030 and 115.4 million by 2050. The sharpest increase in numbers in the incidence of AD is likely to occur in the low and middle income countries. Alexander Roy the chairperson of ARDSI, India and the chairperson of the study "The Dementia India Report 2010" stated in an interview with the newspaper Hindu, Chennai, on April 21, 2011 that in 20 years the number of elderly in India is going to double which will make India the country with the largest number of elderly in the world. The population of 80 year olds is on the increase and thus the increase in the AD population. The prevalence of AD in India is 1/20 in the 60 year olds and 1/5 over 80 year olds. Roy stated that ₹ 3.7 crore Indians are affected by AD and the cost is estimated to be ₹ 14700 crore.

This is going to treble in the next 20 years as the number of affected is going to double to the tune of ₹ 7.6 crore. Much of this increase in AD will be due to aging population in emerging developing countries. More than 50 per cent of people with AD live in developing countries and by 2025 this percentage will be over 70 per cent.

INDIA GUIDE: Population of India 2012 gives the following statistics.

Current: 1,22,200,000 (1.22 billion), Male: 628.8 million. Female: 591.4 million.

Population in 2011 was 1.21 billion, in 2010, 1.02 billion and in 1947 was 350 million.

Alzheimer's Disease International December 2008

Table 1: ADI consensus estimates for the prevalence of dementia (%), by WHO region and age group.

The letters in brackets refer to the level of development of the region; A = lowest mortality regions; E = highest mortality resions.

WHO region	Description	60-64	65-69	70-74	75-79	80-84	85+
EURO (A)	W Europe	0.9	1.5	3.6	6.0	12.2	24.8
EURO (B)	E Europe	0.9	1.3	3.2	5.8	12.2	24.7
EURO (C)	E Europe	0.9	1.3	3.2	5.8	11.8	24.5

WHO region	Description	60-64	65-69	70-74	75-79	80-84	85+
AMRO (A)	N America	0.8	1.7	3.3	6.5	12.8	30.1
AMRO (D)	S America	0.8	1.7	3.4	7.6	14.8	33.2
AMRO (C)	S America	0.7	1.5	2.8	6.2	11.1	28.1
EMRO (B)	Middle East	0.9	1.8	3.5	6.6	13.6	25.5
EMRO (D)	N Africa, Middle East	1.2	1.9	3.9	6.6	13.9	23.5
WPRO (A)	Japan, Australia, NZ	0.6	1.4	2.6	4.7	10.4	22.1
WPRO (B)	China and neighbors	0.6	1.7	3.7	7.0	14.4	26.2
SEARO (B)	Indonesia, SL, Thailand	1.0	1.7	3.4	5.7	10.8	17.6
SEARO (D)	India and neighbors	0.4	0.9	1.8	3.7	7.2	14.4
AFRO (D)	Sub-Saharan Africa	0.3	0.6	1.3	2.3	4.3	9.7
AFRO (E)	Sub-Saharan Africa	0.5	1.0	1.9	3.8	7.0	14.9

Copied from Alzheimer's Disease, International December 2008.

The prevalence of dementia worldwide: Alzheimer's Disease International estimates that there are currently 30 million people with dementia in the world, with 4.6 million new cases annually (one new case every seven seconds). The number of people affected will be over 100 million by 2050. These estimates were derived from detailed population-based studies of the prevalence of dementia in different regions.

Alzheimer's Disease International Work on the Global Prevalence of Dementia

Alzheimer's Disease International in December 2008 reported the trend for lower prevalence of dementia in developing as opposed to developed countries was supported by the consensus judgment of the expert panel, reviewing all available epidemiological data, at least for the least-developed regions in Africa and South Asia. This difference is unexplained merely by shorter survival of people with dementia, as incidence rates are also much lower than those reported in developed countries. Some of the reasons for this are due to mild dementia that is ignored in developing countries because of cultural differences and lower levels exposure to risk factors for dementia such as smoking and cardiovascular disease. Also, in very poor countries few people survive beyond 65 years of age. However, it seems probable that as patterns of morbidity and mortality coverage with those of developed countries, so will dementia prevalence leading to an increased burden of dementia in poorer countries. Even now, most people with dementia live in developing countries; 60 per cent in 2001 rising to 71 per cent by 2040 (Alzheimer's Diseases International December, 2008). On July 16, 2013, University of Cambridge published results from two major cohort studies, revealing that the number of people with dementia in the UK is substantially lower than expected because overall prevalence in the 65 and over age group dropped. Dementia prevalence figures in the UK show decline over past 20 years. Overall prevalence has gone down by 1.8 per cent to an estimated 6.5 per cent of the population. Using the current age profiles of the UK, this corresponds to an estimated 670,000 people over the age of 65 living with dementia, a reduction of more than 20 per cent in the number of people projected to have dementia today compared with 20 years ago. International Alzheimer's Disease Conference 2014 theme was "early detection, treatment and prevention of dementia: Patients' and caregivers perspective."

The latest figures from the follow up study, CFAS 11 (cognitive function and ageing studies) show that there is variation in the proportion of people with dementia across differing areas of deprivation, suggesting that health inequalities during life may influence a person's likelihood of developing dementia.

Prevalence of dementia in women remains higher than men, with 7.7 per cent of women over 65 estimated to have dementia, compared with 4.9 per cent of men. Although the overall prevalence of dementia has fallen, the prevalence of dementia among people living in care homes has increased from 56 per cent of care home residents twenty years ago to 70 per cent today.

The Dementia India Report 2010 was conducted by a team of Indian doctors to study the pattern of incidence of AD throughout India. The team used Mini Mental Status Examination (MMSE) and COMDEX Schedule (Cambridge

Mental Disorder for the elderly EXAM) to make diagnosis of Dementia of Alzheimer's Type.

Men and women are equally at risk to suffer from AD. Those with higher education are at lower risk. India Report 2010 revealed that there is a slight difference in the incidence of AD between East and West of India with lower incidence in East. Mumbai and Northern state of Haryana reported low rates among people who are 60 years of age and older ranging from 1 per cent in rural north India; the lowest reported in the world to 2.7 in urban Chennai. According to this study, the highest incidence is reported in Kerala. The aim of this study was to establish the prevalence and incidence of Alzheimer's disease in India.

The low incidence reported from Haryana in India and Ibadan in Nigeria raises the possibility of environmental factors or gene-environment interactions in the causation of Alzheimer's disease.

The Dementia India Report 2010 reported the following "State-wise estimates the number of Persons with Dementia (PwD) in India."

State-wise estimates were made using meta-analyzed prevalence estimation for India and the 2001 Census data for future projection (Census, 2006). The projected number of people aged 65 and older with dementia for years 2011, 2016 and 2026, varied by state and region in India and corresponding variability in number of people with dementia was also observed. The percentage change in dementia between the base year 2006 and each of the subsequent time periods was calculated. By 2026, more than 500,000 older PwD are expected to be living in Uttar Pradesh and Maharashtra, Rajasthan, Gujarat, Bihar, West Bengal, Madhya Pradesh, Odisha, Andhra Pradesh, Karnataka, Kerala and Tamil Nadu. Around 20,000 to 40,000 PwD are expected within the next 26 years.

Compared to 2006, Delhi, Bihar and Jharkhand are expected to experience 200 per cent or greater increment in total number of dementia cases over the 26 year period. Other states, Jammu and Kashmir, Uttar Pradesh, Rajasthan, Madhya Pradesh, West Bengal, Assam, Chhattisgarh, Gujarat, Andhra Pradesh, Haryana, Uttarakhand, Maharashtra, Karnataka and Tamil Nadu, are estimated to experience over 100 per cent change in number of people who are older. The increased numbers of PwD will have a marked impact on the states' infrastructure and healthcare systems, which are at present ill prepared in many states of India. The projected increase of PwD in the Southern regions is not as marked as those in other regions of India. However, large proportion of people aged 65 would result in greater number of PwD.

REFERENCES

Alexander Roy. ARDSI, Dementia India Report 2010.

Alzheimer's Disease International December 2008. ADI Consensus estimates for the prevalence of Dementia (%) by WHO region and age group.

Alzheimer's Association 2012. Alzheimer's Disease Facts and Figures 2012.

Dementia India Report 2010. "ADI consensus estimates for the prevalence of dementia."

——. "State-wise estimates the number of Persons with Dementia (PwD) in India."

G8 summit in London 2013. Conference on Alzheimer's.

McKhann 1984. NINCDS-ADRDA Alzheimer's Criteria.

Perry George 1995. Alzheimer's by Wikipedia.

Prevalence ARDSI: Facts and Figures 2010.

Teixeira 1995. "Clinico-Pathological Correlation in Dementias." *Journal of Psychiatry and Neuroscience*, 20 (1995): 276-82.

University of Cambridge July 16, 2013: Results from two major cohort studies show that dementia in UK is substantially lower than expected.

2

Historical Background, Conceptual Perspective and Risk Factors

Alzheimer's disease can damage several areas of the brain, and the damage gets progressively worse the longer a person lives with this disorder. The disease was first identified in 1906 by the German psychiatrist Alois Alzheimer. August Deter a 51-year old was his patient who manifested strange behavioral symptoms, including loss of short-term memory. Deter died in April 1906. Alzheimer used the staining techniques to identify amyloid plaques and neurofibrillary tangles. He found that brain damage leads to not only one of the most recognized symptoms of memory loss in Alzheimer's disease, but also damage leads to problems with behavior, depression, and other mental disorders. Other features noted are disturbances of sleep and 'cognitive' functions such as attention, concentration, thinking, judgment and decision-making. He reported on a second case of Johann F., as 'plaque-only' Alzheimer's disease. This statement was based on neuro-histopathology. After very careful analysis, it is concluded that Plaque only cases are also an integrative part of the modern Alzheimer's disease concept (Möller, HJ1, Graeber, M.B. 1998). While everyone who ages experiences loss of brain grey matter, this is normally less than 1 per cent per year. For people with Alzheimer's disease this can occur at a rate of between 3 to 9 per cent per year, and some people show up to 50 per cent loss by the time they get a diagnosis of Alzheimer's.

Historically, George Gleanor a neuropathologist, at University of California isolated a beta protein from human amyloid plaques in 1984. Masters and Beyreuther made antibodies to the ADI's plaque protein, which came to be known as amyloid beta (A-beta). In 1988, they found that A-beta plaques were common and widespread in some elderly people and even detected A-beta in neurologically healthy middle-aged people. Hence, they believed that there is a slow accumulation of A-beta plaques throughout the brain. The symptoms appear only in the late decade of the disease. These authors found that the A-beta protein is a fragment of a much larger neuronal membrane protein called amyloid precursor protein or APP which is prevalent in down syndrome. They reported that A-beta is a toxic agent that causes Alzheimer's disease. In 1990, they questioned the A-beta hypothesis since they appeared well before the onset of dementia. Initially, the authors believed that the tau-based tangles correlated better with dementia. Finally, George Gleanor and Masters and Beyreuther agreed that both of them contribute to AD.

For AD there has long been circumstantial evidence, that a build-up of A-beta aggregation over decades eventually triggers tau aggregation. This represents the last, lethal stage of disease (Li QX et al., 1990).

NEURONS

To understand what AD is, it is necessary to understand the neurons and their functions. The brain and the rest of the nervous system are composed of several different types of cells, but the primary functional unit is a cell called the neuron.

Neuron or nerve cell is an electrically excitable cell that processes and transmits information through electrical and chemical signals. These signals between neurons occur via synapses, specialized connections with other cells. Neurons can connect to each other to form neural networks. Neurons are the core components of the nervous system, which includes the brain, spinal cord and the ganglia of the peripheral nervous system (PNS) which comprises the central nervous system (CNS).

All sensations, movements, thoughts, memories and feelings are the result of signals that pass through neurons. Neurons have three parts: (1) Cell body contains the nucleus. (2) Dendrites branch out and receive messages from other nerve cells. (3) Signals then pass from the dendrites through the cell body and may travel away from the cell body down an axon to another neuron, a muscle cell or cells in some other organ. Axons carry messages from one cell to another in the cortex. Axon may be short or long. Long ones carry messages from the brain to all the way down the spinal cord. The synapse is where the signal passes from the neuron to another cell. The synapse is a structure that permits a neuron (or a nerve cell) to pass an electrical or chemical signal to another cell. When the signal reaches the end of the axon, it stimulates tiny sacs. These sacs release chemicals known as neurotransmitters. There are many neurotransmitters. Neurotransmission or synaptic transmission is communication between neurons as accomplished by the movement of chemicals or electrical signals across a synapse." (Kendra Cherry about education and Wikipedia encyclopedia.) The latter has a very extensive note on neurons. Some studies suggest that AD is a multiple neurotransmitter system disorder (Arai et al., 1992). They suggested that acetyltransferase and acetylcholinesterase are present in AD as opposed to controls without dementia. Neurons do not function in isolation, but in close collaboration with blood vessels and glial cells, which support and protect brain cells. Like neurons, glial cells and blood vessels show changes in structure and function in both Alzheimer's disease and normal aging. An important function that astrocytes perform is to protect neurons against damage by free radicals. Communication between neurons and astrocytes is changed in Alzheimer's disease. These alterations can contribute to synaptic malfunction and synaptic loss, causing cognitive deficits. AD interferes with the proper functioning of neurons and synapses. The accumulation of beta-amyloid is believed to interfere with the neuron to neuron communication at synapses and contributes to cell death. The tau tangles block the transport of nutrients and other essential molecules in the neuron and are also believed to contribute to cell death.

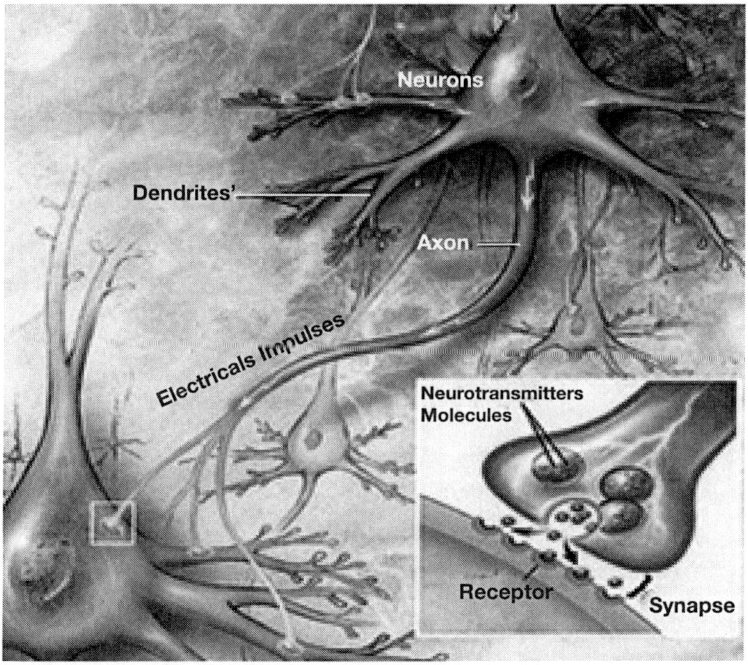

Neuron and neurotransmitter molecule.

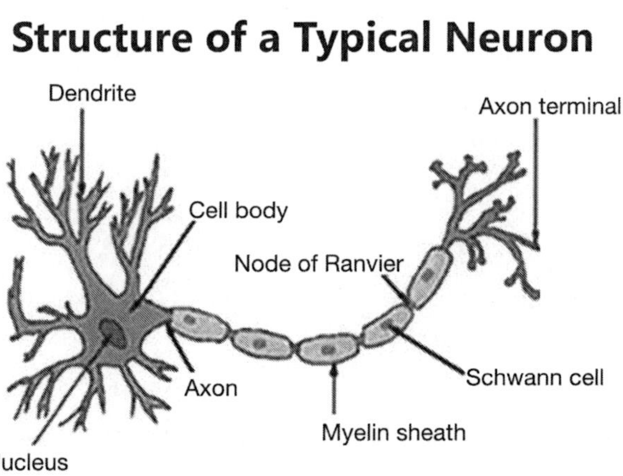

Source: Wikipedia encyclopedia copy

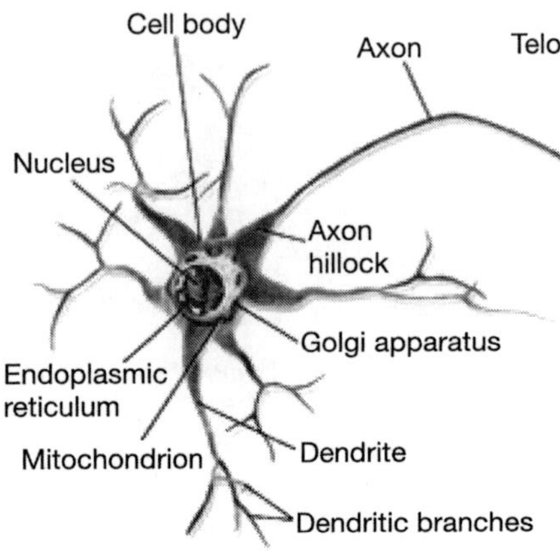

Anatomy of a multipolar neuron.

Source: Wikipedia encyclopedia

Scientists have identified three major categories of neurotransmitters in the human brain.

Biogenic Amine Neurotransmitters

Six main ones are: Serotonin, Norepinephrine, Epinephrine, Dopamine, Histamine, and Acetylcholine. Acetylcholine is supposed to be associated with muscle activation, learning and memory. Alzheimer's type dementia has been linked to acetylcholine function (Neuroscience on line Jack C. Waymire).

Biogenic amines can be found in all foods containing proteins or free amino acids and are found in a wide range of food products including fish products, meat products, dairy products, wine, beer, vegetables, fruits, nuts and chocolate (Wikipedia encyclopedia).

Peptide neurotransmitters is associated with schizophrenia, eating disorders, Huntington's disease and Alzheimer's disease.

Amino Acid Neurotransmitters

They are the main players in the neurotransmission process and they are: 1. Gamma-aminobutyric acid (GABA) is a major inhibitory neurotransmitter that acts through a negative feedback system to block the transmission of a signal from one cell to another cell. 2. Glutamate is important for learning and memory. In Alzheimer's disease, too much of this can cause brain cell death (Wikipedia.org.).

Neurofibrillary Tangle

Neurofibrillary tangles are abnormal structures, composed of twisted masses of protein fibers within nerve cells, found in the brains of people with Alzheimer's disease. In Alzheimer's Disease direct damage to the Neurons occur, through the formation of 'Neurofibrillary Tangles' (NFTs) composed of a protein called 'Tau'. Tau is normally involved in retaining the structure of neurons, however in Alzheimer's disease strands of this protein become tangled together in pairs. This feature first occurs at the ends of the neurons. Then, these chemicals are carried to neighboring cells, and progressively the chemicals spread to more cells. Eventually the neuron's ability to create new signals will weaken and may die. The neurons are the main processing cells in the brain [*Eur Neurol.* 1998 Oct, 40(3): 130-40 and translated by Brion, J.P. and Wikipedia encyclopedia].

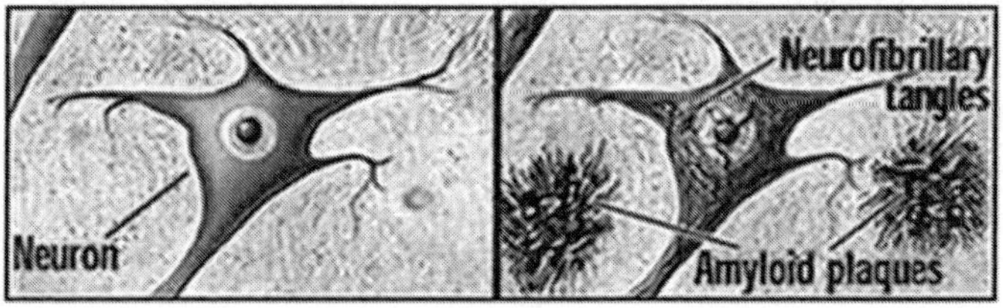

Source: Copy from Wikipedia encyclopedia

PLAQUE

The neuritic plaque is an extracellular deposit consisting of beta-amyloid protein mixed with branches of dying nerve cells which is seen in the brain of a patient with Alzheimer's disease. Neuritic plaques are located outside of the cells and are mainly composed of materials called beta-amyloid and apolipoprotein E (ApoE). Beta-amyloid comes from a protein thought to play a role in neuronal function, and ApoE is involved in neuronal repair. The plaques themselves may not actually damage the brain. Beta amyloid and ApoE are found in majority of people as they age. They may trigger local inflammation that can harm many cells around in that area. Reportedly, there is reduced production of acetylcholine, norepinephrine, serotonin and somatostatin as people age (Ksiezak-Reading H.; Morgan, K. et al., 1994) and National Institute of Health, National Institute of Aging.

Pathological and biological assessment of AD show significant changes in the structure and function of the brain. In Autopsies, the brain reveals presence of neuritic plaques and neurofibrillary tangles that contribute to further deterioration of the brain functions. These factors are accompanied by Granulovascular change, atrophy, cell loss, and ventricular dilation. Neurofibrillary changes are noted throughout the brain. These factors affect Frontal Lobe, Temporal, Parietal and Occipital Lobes. In addition, the Limbic system containing Hippocampus and Amygdala are also affected. The latter is considered to be the seat of memory functions. The tangles and plaques have a strong presence in Hippocampus, Amygdala and other parts of the Limbic system.

AETIOLOGY/RISK FACTORS IN ALZHEIMER'S

The cause for most Alzheimer's cases is still essentially unknown (October 2011 Alzheimer's Association), except for 1 per cent to 5 per cent of cases where genetic differences have been identified. Several theories have been postulated to explain the causes of the disease. Alzheimer's Association stated on October 1, 2011 "What we know about Alzheimer's disease. While scientists know Alzheimer's disease involves progressive brain cell failure, the reason cells fail isn't clear."

Old Age

The biggest risk factor for Alzheimer's disease is old age. Age and genetics are the best-known risk factors for Alzheimer's disease. Aging may be a consistent risk factor in AD this may be due to either an earlier loss of neuronal redundancy or damage to critical neuronal systems exacerbated by environmental exposures across the life-span. After 80/85 of age the risk of AD is about 50 per cent. A person's early life history can also influence Alzheimer's disease risk. For example, studies in 2011 by National Institute of Aging, added to an increasing body of evidence that more years of high school and college education are associated with reduced risk of cognitive decline in old age, and that more years of education may be particularly protective for certain socio-economic groups.

The researchers at the University of California, Berkeley, found a significant association between higher levels of mental stimulation over a lifetime and lower levels of amyloid in the brains of the healthy older volunteers. The relationship remained significant even when accounting for age, gender, and years of education. Other lifetime activities examined such as current levels of cognitive activity, did not show an association with amyloid deposits. The results may suggest frequent engagement in cognitive activity in early and mid-life might help to delay or prevent the abnormal levels of amyloid in the brain, which accompany Alzheimer's disease in later life (Landau, S.M. et al., 2012). The NIA (National Institute of Aging) and the Alzheimer's Association funded the study.

Brain neurons have a remarkable capacity to remodel their connections with other neurons in response to changes in the environment. This phenomenon, known as "synaptic plasticity," is critical for memory processes and for behavioral adaptation to changes in the environment. However, Mt. Sinai Medical Centre, New York City, researchers found that in rats, the remodeling capacity of neurons diminishes with age in the prefrontal cortex, a brain region involved in learning and memory (Bloss, et al.; "Understanding the Biology of Alzheimer's Disease and Aging Brain").

The likelihood of developing Alzheimer's disease doubles every 5.5 years from 65 to 85 years of age. Whereas only 1 per cent to 2 per cent of individuals 70 years of age have Alzheimer's disease, in some studies around 40 per cent of individuals 85 years of age have Alzheimer's disease. Nonetheless, at least half of people who live past the 95 years of age do not have Alzheimer's disease. This was reported by Medicine Net.com.

Cholinergic Hypothesis

The cholinergic hypothesis (Francis, P.T., Snape, M. and Wilcox, G.K., 1999) states that AD is caused by reduced synthesis of the neurotransmitter acetylcholine. This leads to the loss of communication among certain nerve cells and the eventual destruction of these nerve cells. Neurons signal to each other via chemicals called neurotransmitters. The main neurotransmitter that is lost in Alzheimer's disease is known as Acetylcholine. Many of the medications used to help slow the symptoms of AD work by enhancing the levels of this neurotransmitter. Acetylcholine is involved in many aspects of memory, learning, problem-solving and judgment, as well as some aspects of behavior (Francis, P.T., Snape, M. and Wilcox, G., 1999). This hypothesis has not received much support from the scientists community because medications to treat acetylcholine deficiency have not been very effective.

Other neurotransmitters can also be affected in people with AD. For example, memory problems have been linked to the loss of neurons containing Glutamate. Glutamate is a useful excitatory neurotransmitter of the nervous system, although excessive amounts in the brain can lead to cell death through the process called excitotoxicity, which consist of the over stimulation of glutamate receptors. In addition, behavioral problems in people with AD have been linked to loss of neurons containing Dopamine. Dopamine has a number of important functions in the brain, this includes regulation of motor behavior, pleasures related to motivation and also emotional arousal. Depressive symptoms are attributed to the loss of neurons containing Norepinephrine and sleep problems are attributed to the loss of neurons containing Serotonin.

Amyloid Hypothesis

Among the brain changes believed to contribute to the development of AD are the accumulation of the protein Beta-Amyloid outside in the brain and the accumulation of the protein TAU inside neurons each with long branching extensions. In AD, the accumulation of beta-amyloid outside neurons is believed to interfere with the neuron-to-neuron communication of synapses and to contribute to cell death. Inside the neuron, abnormally high levels of Tau form tangles that block the transport of nutrients and other essential molecules throughout the cell. This process is also believed to contribute to cell death. Brains from people with advanced AD show dramatic shrinkage from cell loss and widespread debris from dead and dying neurons. The plaques and tangles can lead to a gradual loss of connections between brain cells and eventually cell death (Tiraboschi, P. et al., 2004).

Amyloid Hypothesis gives a central role to abnormal processing of Amyloid precursor protein—APP—, a certain protein found widely throughout the body but whose normal functions remain unknown. Beta-amyloid is chemically sticky and builds plaques. In Alzheimer's disease, an unknown process causes APP to be divided into smaller fragments by enzymes through proteolysis (Turner, P.R. et al., 2003). One of these fragments gives rise to fibrils of beta-amyloid, which form clumps that deposit outside neurons in dense formations known as senile plaques. The small clumps of Beta-amyloids may block cell-to-cell signaling at synapses. They may also activate immune system cell that trigger inflammation and destroy disabled cells.

Amyloid-beta is formed from a large protein called amyloid precursor protein (APP) (Andrew, Rosenzweig, MD., 2011). Researchers don't exactly know the function of APP yet, but it may impact the activity of brain cells. Special enzymes called secretases cut this protein at specific sites, and one of the products of this "clevage" is the amyloid-beta peptide. These amyloid-beta peptides clump together into what's called oligomers, and according to the amyloid cascade hypothesis, it is these oligomers that are toxic to brain cells, causing the very early cognitive problems in Alzheimer's disease. Later, these oligomers form the plaques that are characteristic of Alzheimer's disease, but it is the oligomers as opposed to the plaques that are the actual toxic agents.

While several lines of evidence that support the amyloid cascade hypothesis, there are also a number of challenges to it (Andrew, Rosenzweig, MD., 2011). For one thing, the Amyloid-beta that accumulates in plaques occurs in normal aging as well as Alzheimer's disease. For another deposits of another protein called Tau form tangles that correlate better with cognitive problems in Alzheimer's disease than do plaques. Finally, there are other alternative theories such as the mitochondrial cascade hypothesis, that have been proposed as explanations of what causes Alzheimer's disease.

The Amyloid hypothesis postulated that beta-amyloid deposits are the fundamental cause of the disease (Hardy, J. and Allsop, D., 1991). Mudher, A. Lovestone in 2002 commenting on Alzheimer's disease asked "do Tauists and Baptists finally shake hands?"

Support for this postulate comes from the location of the gene for the amyloid precursor protein (APP) on chromosome 21, together with the fact that people with trisomy 21 (Down Syndrome) who have an extra gene copy almost universally exhibit AD at 40 years of age (Nistor, M., 2007).

Ne Lott, I.T. and Head, E. (2005) wrote on the topic of Alzheimer Disease and Down Syndrome Factors in pathogenesis. Lott suggested that a specific isoform of apolipoprotein, APOE4, is the main genetic risk factor for AD. Whilst apolipoproteins enhance the breakdown of beta-amyloid, some isoforms are not very effective at this task such as APOE4, leading to excess amyloid build up in the brain (Polvikoski, T., 1995). In 2009, it is theorized that a close relative of the beta-amyloid protein and not necessarily the beta-amyloid itself may be the cause of AD. Further evidence comes from the finding that transgenic mice that express a mutant form of the human APP gene develop fibrillary amyloid plaques and Alzheimer's-like brain pathology with spatial learning deficits (Games, D., 1995).

Recent study revealed that butyrlcholinestrase (BCHE) gene had greater amounts of amyloid. The effect of BCHE was independent of the APOE gene variant. "However both gene variants had more amyloid deposition than those with a single suspect gene" (Ramanan, V.K. et al., 2013).

Family history: Individuals who have a parent, brother or sister with AD are more likely to develop the disease than those who do not have a first-degree relative with AD. Those who have more than one first-degree relative with AD are at even higher risk of developing the disease. When diseases run in families, hereditary (genetics) shared environmental/lifestyle factors or both may play a role.

One known cause of AD is genetic mutation. One per cent of AD is caused by three genetic mutations. They are: gene from the amyloid precursor protein and the genes for the presenilin 1 and 2 proteins. Inheriting any of these genetic mutations guarantees that an individual will develop AD. In such individuals, the disease tends to develop before age 65, sometimes in individuals as young as age 30 known as younger onset or early-onset AD (Waring, S.C. and Rosenberg, R.N. *Arch Neurol.* 2008; 65(3):329-34.) Most of the cases of Alzheimer's disease do not exhibit autosomal-dominant inheritance and are termed sporadic AD. Nevertheless genetic differences may act as risk factors. The best-known genetic risk factor is the inheritance of the 4 allele of the apolipoprotein E (APOEe4). Scientists know genes are involved in Alzheimer's. There are two types of genes that can play a role in affecting whether a person develops a disease—risk genes and deterministic genes. Alzheimer's genes have been found in both categories.

The risk gene with the strongest influence is called apolipoprotein E-e4 (APOE-e4). Scientists estimate that APOE-e4 may be a factor in 20 to 25 per cent of Alzheimer's cases. Deterministic genes directly cause a disease, guaranteeing that anyone who inherits them will develop the disorder. Scientists have discovered variations that directly cause Alzheimer's disease in the genes coding three proteins: amyloid precursor protein (APP), presenilin-1 (PS-1) and presenilin-2 (PS-2).

In October 2013, an international group of researchers reported on the identification of 11 new genes that offer important new insights into the disease pathways involved in Alzheimer's disease. The new genes are: (HLA-DRB5/HLA0DRB1, PTK2B, SLC24A4-0RING3, DSG2, INPP5D, MEF2C, NME8, ZCWPW1, CELF1, FERMT2 and CASS4) add to a growing list of gene variants associated with onset and progression of late-onset Alzheimer's. Genetic risk factors alone are not enough to cause the late-onset form of Alzheimer's disease, so researchers are actively exploring education, diet and environment to learn what role they might play in the development of this disease.

Most experts believe that additional genes may influence the development of late-onset Alzheimer's. Scientists around the world are searching for these genes, and have identified a number of common genes in addition to APOE 4 that may increase a person's risk for late-onset Alzheimer's.

TAU THEORY

Tau is a protein that helps organize and stabilize cell's internal skeleton in AD. The Tau hypothesis is the idea that Tau protein abnormalities initiate the disease cascade (Mudher, A., et al., 2002). Tau theory postulates that it is a protein that helps organize and stabilize cell's internal 'skeleton' in AD. In AD Tau forms and loses its ability to support the cell. Eventually, this leads to Neurofibrillary Tangles which is supposed to be the salient feature of AD. Tangles destroy a vital cell transport system made of proteins. Protein called "Tau" helps the tracks stay straight. In areas where tangles are forming, the Tau collapses into twisted strands called tangles; the tracks can no longer stay straight. They fall apart and disintegrate. Nutrients and other essential supplies can no longer move through the cells, which eventually dies.

This theoretical model of Tau believes that hyper-phosphorylated tau begins to pair with other threads of tau. Eventually, they form neurofibrillary tangles inside nerve cell bodies (Goedert, M. et al., 1991). When this occurs microtubules disintegrate, collapsing the neuron's transport system made of proteins (Iqbal, K. 2005). This may result first in malfunctions in biochemical communication between neurons. Nutrients and other essential supplies can no longer move through the cells and this leads later in the death of the cells and (Chun, W. and Johnson, G.V., 2007). Cleavage in Neuronal Cell Death (Goedert, M., Spillantini, M.G., Crowther, R.A., 1991).

How Tau Pathology Spreads in the Alzheimer's Brain

Neurofibrillary tangles are strong indicators of Alzheimer's disease. Tangles are composed of misfolded forms of the protein tau—a structural change that results in tau clumping into insoluble fibrils. Under the microscope, the tangles resemble thread like fibers that cause tau to misfold and lose function. As Alzheimer's disease progresses, tau pathology spreads from one brain region to another in a consistent pattern. Tangles appear first in the entorhinal cortex, next in the hippocampus, and then in the cerebral cortex. These brain regions are connected to one another via synapses that create communication networks. How tau pathology may spread in the Alzheimer's brains is reported in "Understanding the Biology of Alzheimer's Disease and the Aging Brain" sponsored by National Institute on Aging (2011-2012).

Compared to neurons made from skin cells of cognitively normal volunteers, neurons made from Alzheimer's volunteers showed Alzheimer's-like features, including high levels of abnormal tau as well as beta-amyloid. In addition to development of this important model, the researchers found evidence that both tau and amyloid pathology may result from abnormal processing of amyloid precursor protein (APP) but develop along different pathways. This finding is of clinical importance, as it suggests that drugs targeting beta-amyloid may not improve tau pathology (National Institute of Heath, National Institute of Aging 2011-2012).

Alzheimer's research at the University of Minnesota, neurosciences hypothesizes "Plaques and tangles are late stage lesions of the disease not the cause of it." Ashe lab is focusing on finding the specific proteins that disrupt memory.

Herpes Simplex Virus Type-1

The Herpes Simplex virus type-1 also been proposed to play a causative role in people carrying the susceptible versions of the APOE gene (Bartzokis, G., 2011, 2007, 2004; Itzhaki, R.F. and Wozniak, M.A. 2008). Such type of research is neither well accepted nor funded for research.

Astrocytes and Blood Vessels in Aging and Alzheimer's Disease

Astrocytes protect neurons and blood vessels. Astrocytes secrete growth factors and generate new neurons. Bernal and Peterson (2011) on the basis of research on rats reported importantly, the brain regions in which these astrocyte changes were seen included parts of the hippocampus, where new neurons are generated. These findings indicate that decreased availability of astrocyte-derived growth factors may contribute to age-related declines in neurogenesis.

Beta-amyloid disrupted astrocytes antioxidant production pathways and simultaneously interfered with the astrocytes' ability to protect neurons against beta-amyloid toxicity (Garg et al., University of Michigan, 2011).

In "Understanding the Biology of Alzheimer's Disease and Aging Brain: National Institute on Aging 2011-2012 Alzheimer's Progress Report", Alexie, Verkhratsky et al. (2011-12) stated that Neurons do not function in isolation, but in close collaboration with blood vessels and glial cells, which support and protect brain cells. Like neurons glial cells and blood vessels show changes in structure and function in both Alzheimer's disease and normal aging. These changes can impair healthy brain function. An important function that astrocytes perform is to protect neurons against damage by free radicals. Communication between neurons and astrocytes is changed in Alzheimer's. These alterations can contribute to synaptic malfunction and synaptic loss, causing cognitive deficits. As these progresses, neuronal death and brain atrophy take place causing severe dementia. Free radicals are highly reactive molecules that can build up inside cells due to aging and other factors and cause cellular damage, a condition known as Oxidative stress. The study is conducted by Genetic Science Learning Center, University of Utah.

Through the use of genetic engineering techniques, University of California, San Diego, researchers created neurons from cultured skin cells of people with familial Alzheimer's disease

(Israel et al., National Institute of Health; National Institute of Aging 2011-2012 Alzheimer's Disease).

New Techniques for Studying Alzheimer's Biology, University of California, San Francisco researchers used a new method called "bioluminescence imaging" to rapidly and non-invasively monitor disease progression in the living brains of Alzheimer's model mice (Watts et al., 2010). The new imaging tool tracks disease-related changes in brain astrocytes, the star-shaped cells that help support brain health. Astrocytes increase in number and express more of a gene called Glial Fibrillary Acidic Protein (GFAP) in Alzheimer's disease.

University of Kentucky, Lexington researchers are interested in finding out how physical exercise influence cognitive health into late life. Research showed that exercise benefits aging glial cells which support and protect neurons and blood vessels (Latimer et al., 2011).

Myelin Breakdown

Bartzokis, G. (August 2011), Bartzokis, Lu-Minz, J. 2007, 2004) reported that Alzheimer's disease may be caused by age-related myelin breakdown in the brain. Iron released during myelin breakdown is hypothesized to cause further damage. Homeostatic myelin repair processes contribute to the development of proteinaceous deposits such as beta-amyloid and tau.

Myelin is a fatty sheath that coats the axons of the nerves, allowing the efficient conduction of nerve impulses. It is responsible for the fast processing speeds that underlie the higher cognitive functioning.

As people age, myelin tends to get damaged. In a report in the journal *Alzheimer's* and *Dementia*, George Bartzokis, UCLA professor of neurology, suggests that it is the breakdown of this late-stage myelin that promotes the building up of toxic amyloid-beta fibrils that eventually deposit in the brain and become the plaques which have long been associated with Alzheimer's disease. These amyloid products in turn destroy more and more myelin, disrupting brain signaling and leading to cell death and the classic clinical signs of Alzheimer's.

Alzheimer's Disease and HSV 1

HSV 1 has been noted as cause for AD (Itzhaki, R.F. and Wozniak, M.A. 2008) (Holmes, C. and Cotterell, D., 2009). In the presence of certain gene variation (APOE-epsilon 4 allele carriers), the virus interacts with the components and receptors of lipoproteins, which may lead to the development of AD (Dobson, C. and Itzhaki, R.F., 1999 and Pyles, R.B. November 2001) without the presence of gene allele HSV type 1 does not appear to cause any neurological damage and thus increase the risk of AD (Itzhaki, R.F. et al., 1997). Herpes simplex virus type 1 DNA is localized within the beta-amyloid plaques that characterize AD (Wozniak, M.A. et al., 2009). It suggests that this virus is a major cause of the plaques and hence probably a significant etiological factor in AD.

Neuro-inflammation and Alzheimer's Pathology

Neuro-inflammation is associated with AD pathology. Neuro-inflammation includes brain cells such as microglia and astrocytis (AChR) both generate beta amyloid protein, one of the main pathological features of AD. Patients taking anti-inflammatory drugs had a lower risk of AD than those who did not. Individuals taking anti-inflammatory drugs to treat such conditions as arthritis appear to have a lower-than-expected occurrence of AD. "Neuro-inflammation is involved in the pathogenesis of neurological diseases and disorder, but its contribution and involvement to the pathological processes remain to be elucidated. It may be involved in the modulation of neurogenesis in neurological diseases and disorders, but the contribution and significance of this modulation remain to be understood. Neuro-inflammation has tremendous implications for cellular therapy" (Taupin, P., 2008) and (McGreer, E.G. and Mcgeer, P.L., 2010).

Inflammation may contribute to the development of dementia in many ways. Inflammation strongly affects risk of CVD. Additionally, microglial activation and acute phase reactants have been noted at typical sites of AD pathology, (Casserly, I. et al., 2004), although this could be an effect rather than a cause of neurological degeneration. Inflammation appears to directly contribute to neuronal dysfunction and death, and mice which over express COX-2 (an enzyme which regulates inflammation) demonstrate increased neuronal susceptibility to toxic insult (Akiyama, H. et al., 2000). Moreover, in transgenic mice, inflammatory proteins induce amyloid beta accumulation and deposition. Finally, in direct studies of memory, mice that over express IL-6 exhibit deficits in learning and memory tasks.

In "Understanding the Biology of Alzheimer's Disease and Aging Brain", the section on Inflammatory and Immune Responses in Alzheimer's and Brain Aging, reported that Alzheimer's brain has signs of continuous inflammation, which is a tissue response to cellular damage. A University of California, Irvine, study suggests that chronic inflammation contributes to neurodegeneration in Alzheimer's disease (Kitazawa et al., 2011). Bell et al. (2012) suggested that APOE gene increases AD risk by setting off an inflammatory response that leads to breakdown of the blood-brain barrier. They further stated that when the blood-brain barrier breaks down, brain blood vessels begin to leak toxic proteins that enter the brain, and neurons degenerate. They further reported that inflammation and blood-barrier breakdown may precede beta-amyloid accumulation in the Alzheimer's disease process.

The use of animal models for Alzheimer's disease research has been useful. However, mouse cells do not act like human cells. The plaques in mice do not exhibit tau tangles. Promising studies, however, have developed new human cellular models for studying Alzheimer's biology. So said one researcher.

ALCOHOL

Strong and consistent evidence indicates that moderate alcohol intake might reduce the risk of cognitive impairment and AD, although higher levels have an adverse effect on brain function. The potential neuroprotection of moderate alcohol most probably is the result of numerous vascular benefits associated with alcohol intake (Stampfer, M.J. et al., 2005).

Epidemiological data regarding the potential impact of antioxidant vitamins on cognitive decline and dementia are mixed. Clear evidence from several randomized clinical trials establishes that short-term use (10 years) of vitamin supplements (Lancet, 2002) does not protect against cognitive impairment, but very long-term use (15+ years) could be neuroprotective. Similarly, there is no consistent evidence that antioxidant supplements decrease the risk of AD, but no studies have specifically addressed long-term use of supplements (Petersen, R.C. et al., 2005).

Plasma Homocysteine was Noted as a Risk Factor for Dementia and Alzheimer's Disease

An increased plasma homocysteine level is a strong, independent risk factor for the development of Alzheimer's. An analysis from the Framingham study has revealed that elevated plasma levels of Homocysteine is a significant risk factor for dementia and Alzheimer's disease. There is an association between high plasma Homocysteine and significant memory loss (Sudha, Sesadri, MD; Alexa, Beiser, Ph.D. et al., 2002).

People with elevated levels of homocysteine in the blood had nearly double the risk of developing Alzheimer's disease, according to a new report from scientists at Boston University. The findings, in a group of people participating in the long-running Framingham study, are the first to tie Homocysteine levels measured several years earlier with later diagnosis of AD and other dementias. The report, which appears in the February 14, 2002, issue of *The New England Journal of Medicine*, provides some of the most powerful evidence yet.

Oxidative Stress and Dys-Homeostasis of Biometal (Biology) Metabolism

The oxidative stress and dys-homeostasis of biometal metabolism may be significant in the formation of pathology (Su B. Wang. et al., 2008) (Kastenholz, B., Grfin, D.E., Horst, J. and Nagel, K.A., 2009). The oxidative stress is the cell damage associated with the chemical reaction between free radicals and other molecules in the body. Major hurdle in understanding AD is a lack of knowledge about the etiology and pathogenesis of selective neuron death. In recent years, considerable data have accrued indicating that the brain in AD is under increased oxidative stress and this may have a role in the pathogenesis of neuron degeneration and death in this disorder. The direct evidence supporting increased oxidative stress in AD is: (i) increased brain Fe (Iron), Al (Aluminum), and Hg (Mercury) in AD, capable of stimulating free radical generation; (ii) increased lipid peroxidation and decreased polyunsaturated fatty acids in the AD brain, and increased 4-hydroxynonenal, an aldehyde product of lipid peroxidation in AD ventricular fluid; (iii) increased protein and DNA oxidation in the AD brain; (iv) diminished energy metabolism and decreased cytochrome c oxidase in the brain in AD; (v) advanced glycation end products (AGE), malondialdehyde, carbonyls, peroxynitrite, heme oxygenase-1 and SOD-1; and (vi) studies showing that amyloid-beta peptide are capable of generating free radicals (Markesbery, W.R., 1997).

Type-2 Diabetes and Alzheimer's

A research team in Israel has devised a novel approach to identifying the molecular basis for designing a drug that might one day decrease the risk diabetic patients face of developing Alzheimer's disease. The team recently presented its work at the 57th Annual Meeting of the Biophysical Society (BPS) in Philadelphia, on February 2-6, 2013.

A recent study suggests that people who suffer from type-2 diabetes face twice the risk of developing Alzheimer's disease later in life compared to those who do not have diabetes. The link these diseases share relates to the formation of two types of peptide deposits that aggregate, or clump together. Peptides are chains of amino acids; longer chains form proteins. One type of peptide, called amyloid beta, is found in Alzheimer plaques in neurons of the brain. The other type, myelin, is found in the pancreas and the brain. Two years ago, researchers found both molecules in the pancreas of diabetic patients, and in both diseases their presence has been linked to the progression of the disease state.

Mount Sinai of Medicine researchers have found that a gene associated with onset of Type-2 diabetes is also found at lower than normal levels in people with AD. There seems to be a relationship between Type-2 and onset of progression of AD. Research headed by Ginlio, Maria Pasinetti, MD, Ph.D. Professor of Psychiatry and Geriatrics at Mount Sinai School of medicine in October 2010, said: "The relationship between type-2 diabetes and Alzheimer's disease is elusive, not all subjects with type-2 diabetes are affected by Alzheimer's disease and similarly, not all Alzheimer's disease cases are diabetic." However, in the last few years, epidemiological evidence indicates that relative to healthy elderly subjects, people of the same age affected by type-2 diabetes are twice as likely to develop Alzheimer's disease. The reason is not known. The new study from Dr. Pasinetti, reported in this week's issue of Archives of Neurology, provides insight into a potential mechanism that might explain the relationship between type-2 diabetes and Alzheimer's disease, onset and progression (Ginlio Maria Pasinetti, MD, 2009). A few researchers believe that Alzheimer's disease is a third form of diabetes. They believe that a toxic protein found in the brains of AD is a form of diabetes. Some researchers think that Alzheimer's removes insulin receptors from nerve cells, rendering those neurons insulin resistant. North Western University researchers term AD as being a "type-3 diabetes" (I do not think individuals who suffer from diabetes should be alarmed by this theory since no definite conclusion is reached). The protein known to attack memory-forming synapses is called ADDL for 'Amyloid B-derived diffusible ligand'. Drugs now used to improve insulin may protect neurons from ADDLs. (This study needs further research. As such this is anxiety evoking for those who suffer from diabetes.)

Depression

Depressive symptoms are risk factors in AD. Alzheimer's and depression may manifest simultaneously. Depression by itself may not suggest Alzheimer's as reported by Martha Storandt, Gary R. VandenBos, 1995, in *Dementia and Depression.*

Early Alzheimer's disease and depression share many symptoms, so it can be difficult even for doctors to distinguish between the two disorders. And many people with Alzheimer's also are depressed. One important difference between Alzheimer's and depression is in the effectiveness of treatment. While Alzheimer's drugs can only slow the progression of cognitive decline, medications to treat depression can improve a person's quality of life dramatically.

People who have both Alzheimer's and depression may find it easier to cope with the changes caused by Alzheimer's when they feel less depressed.

Other theories of Alzheimer's in vogue are the following:

CHEMICAL THEORY

John Hopkins University studies accept the chemical theory. It states that there are biochemical changes in the brain and some of the biochemicals are harmful to the brain. One biochemical is known as Nerve Growth FACTOR (NGF).

Nerve growth factor is a small-secreted protein that is important for the growth, maintenance, and survival of certain target neurons (nerve cells).

Researchers are not in agreement as to how much NGF is good since the nervous system of the brain showed nerve death when given too much. John Hopkins University reported of Emerging New Nervous Theory of Allergy on May 19, 2000.

Acetylcholine is effective if given early in the disease process. Chemical theory deals with various different chemicals found in high levels in the brain. They include: aluminum, mercury, lead and other metals found in the brains of many AD patients. There is no agreement among the theorists about these chemicals causing AD (Alzheimer's Part 1 by Sandy Corder, Yahoo Contributor Network December 16, 2008). The AD has diminished levels of various neurotransmitters. Low levels of neurotransmitters are thought to influence intellectual functioning and behavior.

EXCESS OF TOXIC CHEMICALS

Increase deposits of aluminum have been found in ADs brain. Toxic chemical especially environmental chemicals can contribute to neurodegenerative changes. UK/Ireland/Australia scientists have discarded the aluminum theory causing AD. Aluminum exists in the plaques and tangles in the brains of Alzheimer's patients. Some have suggested that aluminum absorption by humans could increase the risk. However, studies have failed to find a link. Aluminum exists in some plants and foods. It is found in some cooking pots and pans, medicines and packaging. Scientists doubt whether there is a link because our bodies absorb minimum amounts and is eliminated from the bodies through the urine.

CHRONIC EXPOSURE OF INDUSTRY WORKERS TO DIACETYL

Although diacetyl forms naturally in fermented beverages such as beer and wine, its chemical structure is similar to a substance that makes beta-amyloid proteins clump together in the brain. This clumping, the study authors noted, is a hallmark of Alzheimer's disease. American Chemical Society reported that diacetyl is used to give a buttery taste to popcorn (Aug. 1, 2012). Diacetyl (DA3) increases the level of beta-amyloid clumping. It enhances beta-amyloid toxic effects on nerve cells growing in laboratory and it easily penetrated the blood-brain barrier. "Butter Flavoring Exposure" is linked to harmful brain process stated Mary Elizabeth Dallas (August 6, 2012). Working with diacetyl may raise risk of proteins clumping in the brain, similar to Alzheimer's. Chronic exposure to an artificial butter flavoring ingredient, known as diacetyl, may worsen the harmful effects of a protein in the brain linked to Alzheimer's disease, according to a new study. The findings should serve as a red flag for factory workers with significant exposure to the food-flavoring ingredient. This was the suggestion by researchers from the University of Minnesota. The report is published in a recent issue of the *Journal of Chemical Research in Toxicology* (August 1, 2012).

Artificial Butter Flavoring Ingredient Linked to Key Alzheimer's Disease Process

A new study raises concern about chronic exposure of workers in industry to a food flavoring ingredient used to produce the distinctive buttery flavor and aroma of microwave popcorn, margarines, snack foods, candy, baked goods, pet foods and other products. It found evidence that the ingredient, diacetyl, intensifies the damaging effects of an abnormal brain protein linked to Alzheimer's disease. The study appears in ACS' *Journal Chemical Research in Toxicology*.

SLOW VIRUS THEORY

Up till now a virus has not been isolated from the brains of AD individuals. The possibility of a viral cause of AD cannot be either eliminated or confirmed.

Because a slow-acting virus has been identified as a cause of some brain disorders that closely resemble Alzheimer's disease, for example, Creutzfeldt-Jakob disease, a slow virus has been postulated in Alzheimer's disease. Various researchers have suggested that suspicious brain tissue changes in Alzheimer's disease may be caused by a virus (Jeri McBride, 2010). However, the virus has not been isolated from the brains of Alzheimer's patients.

The above slow virus theory is not recognized by theorists any more. Now many think that Kuru and Creutzfeldt-Jakob diseases among others can be transmitted by proteinaceous infectious agents or 'prions'. These 'prions' are thought to be natural body proteins that for some reason change their shape, and in so doing induce other proteins to change their shape, messing up the processes of the cell. The prion hypothesis was proposed by Stanley Prusiner, who received a Nobel Prize for this work. "So, I think the reason you aren't hearing much about 'Slow viruses' is that they are no longer a favored scientific theory. The slow virus theory has been replaced by the prion theory." Question answered by Richard, Barrans Jr., Ph.D. Argonne National Labs.

BLOOD VESSEL THEORY

Defects in blood vessels supplying blood to the brain have been studied as possible cause of AD. Hardening of the arteries also known as Cerebroateriosclerosis, proved not to be a cause of AD. Thus, the hyperbaric oxygen chamber treatment produces ineffective as therapy for AD. Some defects and patches in blood vessels supplying blood to neurons can also cause Alzheimer's disease. Evidence does not support the theory one way or the other. Repeated strokes can cause symptoms similar to Alzheimer's. This is called Multi-Infarct Dementia, and strokes occur when fatty deposits narrow arteries in the brain. So blood vessel defects have been studied as a possible cause of Alzheimer's. But so far this line of investigation seems to be a blind alley (Jeri, McBryde. November 2, 2010).

AUTOIMMUNE THEORY

The body's immune system, which protects against potentially harmful foreign invaders, may erroneously begin to attack its own tissues, producing antibodies to its own essential cells. This is called an autoimmune response, and it may take place in the brain. Some scientists speculate that certain late life changes in aging neurons—the major nerve cells of the brain—might be triggering an autoimmune response that evokes symptoms of Alzheimer's disease in vulnerable individuals.

In AD, the immune system of the human body fails and starts to work reversibly. Actually, the immune system of a human body may start attacking its own cells and tissues. Defective cells may be unable to clean up brain plaque in Alzheimer's disease.

"Macrophages are the janitors of the innate immune system, gobbling up waste products in the brain and throughout the body," says study leader (Dr.) Milan Fiala of UCLA. "If further study shows that this defective macrophage function is present in most Alzheimer's disease patients, new hormonal or immune-boosting approaches may offer ways to treat disease."

Age alone cannot be the only cause of AD. Chronic inflammation may lead to neurotoxicity. Polymorphism in pro-inflammatory substances can lead to AD development. A new diagnostic and therapeutic target could be represented by Anti-AB Peptides. Both autoimmunity and inflammation have a role in developing AD.

One of the latest hypotheses is about the role of blood-brain barrier (BBB), as its loss of integrity may lead to a passage of proteins in Cerebro Spinal Fluid (CSF), causing a compromised role of BBB in preserving the brain as an "immune sanctuary". (*Britanica Encyclopedia* on autoimmune theory).

Cardio Vascular Disease Factor and Alzheimer's

Alzheimer's disease is a devastating condition that is increasing in prevalence. No known prevention or cure exists for Alzheimer's disease. Cardiovascular risk factors are prevalent and increase in the elderly, and there have been conflicting reports of associations between modifiable cardiovascular risk factors and Alzheimer's disease. The mechanisms for these associations are uncertain, but they are likely to be the result of a combination of direct and cerebrovascular disease-related mechanisms. From this standpoint, diabetes and hyperinsulinemia seem to have the strongest evidence from laboratory, clinical, and epidemiologic studies. Studies have also indicated that hypertension, hyperlipidemia, hyperhomocysteinemia, and smoking are potentially important risk factors for Alzheimer's disease (Luchsinger, J.A. and Mayeux, R., 2004). They discussed on topic of raising good cardiovascular risk factors and Alzheimer's disease.

Cardiovascular risk factors play an important role in determining the onset of non-genetic AD. Vascular risk factors for AD include stroke, hypertension, diabetes, homocysteine, smoking, hypercholesterolemia, heart failure and atrial fibrillation. It is possible that these can trigger cerebrovascular disease and can precipitate AD.

The health of the brain is closely linked to the overall health of the heart and blood vessels. Healthy blood vessels help ensure that the brain is supplied with oxygen and nutrient-rich blood it needs to function (Stampfer, M.J., 2006).

Evidence supports a strong and likely casual association between cardiovascular disease (CVD) and its risk factors, with incidence of cognitive decline and Alzheimer's. Several cardiovascular risk factors are also risk factors for dementia, including hypertension, high LDL, cholesterol, low HDL cholesterol and especially diabetes.

Several randomized clinical trials have examined the relationship of treatment for high blood pressure to cognitive function and dementia. However, findings have been mixed. The Medical Research Council's trial of hypertension (Stampfer, M.J., 2006) measured performance on two cognitive tests; paired associate learning test and trail making test part A. Amongst 2584 participants aged 65 years and older, there was no difference in the rates of decline on either test for those assigned to antihypertensive.

AD and stroke together account for the bulk of cognitive impairment and mortality worldwide. As the risk factors and causes of stroke are becoming better understood, interventions have started to decrease the incidence of stroke. By contrast, despite three decades of intense research, the etiology of late-onset AD remains to be elucidated, and the incidence of this disease is steadily increasing. The present collection of papers illustrates that progress is being made on several fronts and indicates that many avenues of enquiry remain to be explored (Alan P. Hudson; Brian J. Bali; Keith Crutcher; Stephen Robinson. Published in final edited form as: *Nat Rev Neurol.* 2011 March; 7(3): 137-52).

CHOLESTEROL AND STROKE

Cholesterol levels, diabetes, and hypertension—known risk factors for strokes and heart attacks—can contribute to risk of cognitive decline and dementia later in life. Cholesterol may protect against dementia. One possible explanation for this apparent contradiction may lie in recent research suggesting that an enzyme that breaks down insulin may also have a role in breaking down key abnormal proteins implicated on Alzheimer's disease. "Managing insulin may have a beneficial impact on the brain," said Jacobo Mintzer, a researcher and professor at the Medical University of South Carolina.

"These data help to confirm the idea that cardiovascular health and brain health are closely related. By working to prevent strokes and heart attacks, we may also delay cognitive decline in the elderly," Albert said.

Diabetes drug is effective in early Alzheimer's disease. Recent research has indicated that diabetes may increase the risk for Alzheimer's disease. Some scientists believe that impaired insulin function is the common link between the two diseases. Alzheimer's Association (PR 7-20-2004) reports that some anti-hypertension medicines are associated with reduced risk of Alzheimer's.

Stages of Alzheimer's Disease and Risk Factors

2012 facts and figures published by Alzheimer's association, review the current theories of AD. "The cause or causes of AD are not yet known. The time between the initial brain changes of AD and the symptoms of advance AD is considered by scientist to represent the 'continuum' of AD."

2012 facts and figures by NIA and Alzheimer's association define the different stages of Alzheimer's as follows:

The three stages of Alzheimer's disease proposed by the New Criteria and Guidelines for the Diagnosis of Alzheimer's Disease (Alzheimer's Society and Alzheimer's Association):

(1) Preclinical Alzheimer's disease; (2) mild cognitive impairment (MCI) due to Alzheimer's disease; and (3) dementia due to Alzheimer's disease.

Preclinical Alzheimer's Disease

In this stage, individuals have measurable changes in the brain, cerebrospinal fluid and/or blood (biomarkers) that indicated the earliest signs of disease, but they have not yet established diagnostic criteria that doctors can use now.

Mild Cognitive Impairment (MCI) such as Memory Loss

Individuals with MCI have mild but measurable changes in thinking abilities that are noticeable to the person affected and to family members and friends. The rate of progression for them may be around 10 per cent per year. Only some people with MCI develop dementia. Biomarkers are suggested to diagnose AD. If changes in the brain, cerebrospinal fluid and/or blood, are caused by physiological processes due to AD then diagnosis of MCI due to AD can be made.

MCI is a condition in which individuals have memory problems more often than of the average person of their age. They can still function carrying out the normal activities. People who manifest MCI may often misplace objects, forget events and appointments and may have difficulties to recall words that they want to use in conversations especially if the words are overused ones.

According to the recent research, MCI has been called the transitional state between cognitive changes of normal aging and Alzheimer's disease. Many people who experience mild cognitive impairment are at a high risk of developing Alzheimer's disease. Several studies have indicated that MCI individuals are at an increased risk for developing AD, ranging from 1 per cent to 25 per cent per year; 24 per cent of MCI patients progressed to AD in two years and 20 per cent more over three years, whereas a recent study indicated that the progression of MCI subjects was 55 per cent in four and a half years. Some patients with MCI, however, never progress to AD (Arnaiz, E., Almkvist, O., 2003) and Alzheimer's Society.

Dementia Due to Alzheimer's Disease

This stage is characterized by memory, thinking and behavioral symptoms that impair a person's ability to function in daily life and that are caused by Alzheimer's disease-related processes.

Biomarker Tests:

1. Biomarkers showing the level of beta-amyloid accumulation in the brain.

2. Biomarkers showing that nerve cells in the brain are injured or actually degenerating. Disease modifying treatments will be available in future.

Risk Factors Mentioned by Alzheimer's Association

- Beta-amyloid accumulation outside neuron
- Genetic mutation
- Advanced age
- Family history—genetics
- Apolipoprotein E-e4 (APOE-e4)
- Cardiovascular disease risk factors
- Social engagement and diet
- Head trauma and traumatic brain injury (TBI).

Social engagement and diet: Individuals will have to remain socially and mentally active. Healthy diet for the brain will comprise diet that is low in saturated fats and rich on vegetables. It is not convincingly proved that social engagement or diet may affect AD risk. Findings from a few studies suggest that social engagement and absorbing leisure activities may play a role in maintaining cognitive function in late adulthood and even in delaying or preventing dementia. These studies have largely been correlational in nature, so that it is impossible to know whether people who age gracefully have selected engaged lifestyles or whether those lifestyle behaviors themselves promote healthy aging. Caution is also required in assuming that activities that improve cognitive functioning in older adults who do not have dementia will contribute to preventing AD.

HEAD TRAUMA AND TRAUMATIC BRAIN INJURY (TBI)

"Head injury, head trauma and TBI are associated with an increased risk of Alzheimer's disease and other dementia. Moderate head injuries are associated with twice the risk of developing Alzheimer's compared to no head injuries, and severe head injuries are associated with 4.5 times the risk.

Groups that experience repeated head injuries, such as boxers, football players and combat veterans, may be at increased risk of dementia of late-life cognitive impairment and evidence of tau tangle. Some studies suggest that APOE-e4 carriers who experience moderate or severe head injury are at higher risk of developing Alzheimer's than APOE-e4 carriers who do not have a history of moderate or severe head injury. Additional research is needed to better understand the association between brain injury and increased risk of Alzheimer's" (2012 Alzheimer's disease facts and figures, p. 11).

SLEEP AND MEMORY

Sleep is related to memory. In a study conducted by Turner, Drummond, Salamat, and Brown (2007), working memory was shown to be affected by sleep deprivation. Working memory is important because it keeps information active for further processing and supports higher level cognitive functions like decision-making, reasoning, processing and episodic memory.

These factors are reported in "Understanding the Biology of Disease and Aging Brain 2011-2012"; Alzheimer's Disease Progress Report by National Institute on Aging.

Wikipedia encyclopedia reports the following on sleep and memory. Sleep deprivation, whether it is total sleep deprivation or partial sleep deprivation, can impair working memory in measures of memory, speed of cognitive processing, attention and task switching. Casement et al. found that when subjects were asked to recognize digits displayed on a screen by typing them on a keypad, the working memory speed of subjects whose sleep was restricted to four hours a night (approximately 50 per cent of their normal sleep amount) were 58 per cent slower than control groups who were allowed their full eight hours of sleep.

Neuroplasticity has been thoroughly researched over the past few decades and results have shown that significant changes that occur in the cortical processing areas have the power to modulate neuronal firing to both new and previously experienced stimuli. The changes in quantity of a certain neurotransmitter as well as how the post-synaptic terminal responds to this change are underlying mechanisms of brain plasticity. During sleep there are remarkable changes in modulatory neurotransmitters throughout the brain. Acetylcholine is an excitatory neurotransmitter that is seen to increase to near waking levels during REM sleep while compared to lower levels during slow-wave sleep (Wikipedia, sleep and Memory).

NEURODEGENERATION AND THE AGING BRAIN

Recent neuroimaging studies have shown that 25 to 50 per cent of cognitively normal older adults have significant accumulations of brain beta-amyloid, which may represent an early stage of the Alzheimer's disease process. In a postmortem study led by University of Washington, Seattle researchers, (Sonnen et al., 2011), the brains of many cognitively normal older adults showed signs of other dementia disorders as well. The findings suggest that the brains of a large proportion of cognitively normal people show accumulations of cellular damage, likely the result of one or more diseases or other factors influencing the brain health over life span. These people still enjoy cognitive functions. Researchers will have to find an answer.

MITOCHONDRIAL DYSFUNCTION IN ALZHEIMER'S DISEASE

Mitochondria are the 'powerhouses' of the cell, generating the energy needed to function and survive. In Alzheimer's disease, abnormal levels of beta-amyloid damage brain mitochondria, leading to neuronal dysfunction. A team led by investigators at Columbia University, New York City, found that beta-amyloid interacts with mitochondria by binding to a mitochondrial enzyme called ABAD (beta-amyloid-binding alcohol dehydrogenase) (Yao et al., 2011). "Treating Alzheimer's model mice with a peptide that blocks beta-amyloid binding to ABAD improved mitochondrial function and also alleviated the mice's memory deficits." This study strongly implicates mitochondrial beta-amyloid as a critical player in the development of Alzheimer's disease.

Synapses depend on nearby mitochondria to generate the energy needed for proper functioning. A study led by Harvard University, Cambridge, MA, researchers showed that abnormal forms of tau disrupt this process (Kopeikina et al., 2011). In mice expressing a mutant form of human tau, neurons lacked the mitochondria needed for proper functioning; similar abnormalities were seen at autopsy in people diagnosed with Alzheimer's. The researchers also found that tau does not have to form thread-like fibrils to disrupt mitochondria from delivering energy to synapses. Rather, reduced levels of normal tau in mouse models are enough to disrupt the process.

Katherine, J. Kopeikina et al. find that "tau accumulation cause Mitochondrial Distribution Deficits in Neurons in a Mouse model of Taupathy and in Human Alzheimer's Disease Brain (*The American Journal of Pathology*, Vol. 179, No. 4, October 2011). The Alzheimer's disease brain shows signs of inflammation, a tissue response to cellular damage. In the short-term, inflammation helps neutralize and flush out harmful substances. However, the inflammatory response may damage tissue if it goes on for too long. A University of California, Irvine, study suggests that chronic inflammation contributes to neurodegeneration in Alzheimer's disease (Kitazawa et al., 2011).

Through the use of genetic engineering techniques, University of California, San Diego, researchers created neurons from cultured skin cells of people with familial Alzheimer's disease (Israel et al., 2012) [University of Cambridge Communications (oeac@admin.cam.ac.uk) 22-05-2013 to Jane George].

"Scientist identify molecular trigger for Alzheimer's disease."

For the first time, researchers in the Department of Chemistry have been able to map the pathway from protein malfunction, which lies at the root of Alzheimer's, to neural malfunction. The neurodegenerative process giving rise to diseases such as Alzheimer's is triggered when the normal structures of protein molecules within cells become corrupted.

Amyloid fibrils can form the foundations of huge protein deposits—or plaques—long seen in the brains of Alzheimer's sufferers, and once believed to be the cause of the disease, before the discovery of 'toxic oligomers' by Dobson and others a decade or so ago. A plaque's size and density renders it insoluble, and consequently unable to move. Whereas the oligomers, which give rise to Alzheimer's disease, are small enough to spread easily around the brain-killing neurons and interacting harmfully with other molecules—but how they were formed was until now a mystery.

Dr. Thomas Knowles and collaborators (22-05-2013, University of Cambridge Communications) have now established the pathway that shows how the toxic species that cause cell death, the oligomers, are formed. This is the key pathway to detect, target and intervene—the molecular catalyst that underlies the pathology. "With a disease like Alzheimer's, you have to intervene in a highly specific manner to prevent the formation of the toxic agents. Now we've found how the oligomers are created, we know what process we need to turn off."

(Further more they suggested that Proliferation of amyloid-β42 aggregates occurs through a secondary nucleation mechanism.2013 e-mail communication.)

REFERENCES

Alzheimer's association PR (2004). Some Anti-Hypertension Medicines Associated with Reduced Risk of Alzheimer's, Public release date: 20 Jul.

Alzheimer's Association. Retrieved 1 October 2011: What we know today about Alzheimer's disease.

Alzheimer's diseases Facts and Figures 2012, p. 11: Additional research is needed to better understand the association between brain injury and increased risk of Alzheimer's.

Akiyama, H., Barger S., Barnum S. et al. Inflammation and Alzheimer's disease: Neurobiol Aging 2000; 21: 383–421. *PubMed, CAS*, Web of Science.

Alan P. Hudson, Brian J. Balin, Keith Crutcher, Stephen Robinson. Published in final edited form as: *Nat Rev Neurol.* 2011 March; 7(3): 137–52.

Alexei, Verkhratsky, Markel Olabarria; et al. (2011-2012). National Institute of Aging: Understanding the Biology of Alzheimer's disease and Aging Brain: Astrocytes in Alzheimer's Disease.

American chemical Society August, 1, 2012. Dicetyl is used to give a buttery taste.

ARAI, G. *Lynch Journal Brain Research*. Vol. 598, Nos., 1-2, pp. 173-84, 1992. xx.

Arnáiz, E., and Almkvist, O. (2003). "Neuropsychological features of mild cognitive impairment and preclinical Alzheimer's disease". *Acta Neurol. Scand., Suppl.* 179: 34–41. doi:10.1034/j.1600-0404.107.s179.7.x.

Bartzokis, G., Lu, P.H. and Mintz, J. (December 2004). "Quantifying Age-Related Myelin Breakdown with MRI: Novel Therapeutic Targets for Preventing Cognitive Decline and Alzheimer's Disease". *J. Alzheimer's Dis.* 6 (6 Suppl): S53–9. PMID 15665415

——. (April 2007). "Human Brain Myelination and Beta-amyloid Deposition in Alzheimer's Disease". *Alzheimer's Dement* 3 (2): 122–5. doi:10.1016/j.jalz.2007.01.019. PMC 2442864. PMID 18596894 xx.

Bartzokis, G. (August 2011). "Alzheimer's Disease as Homeostatic Responses to Age-related Myelin Breakdown". *Neurobiol. Aging* 32 (8): 1341–71. doi:10.1016/j.neurobiolaging.2009.08.007. PMC 3128664. PMID 19775776.

Bell et al. (2012). Understanding the Biology of Alzheimer's Disease and Brain Aging. Inflammatory and immune Responses in Alzheimer's and the aging.

Bernal and Peterson (2011). How aging impacts astrocytes. Understanding the Biology of Alzheimer's Disease and the Aging brain. Alzheimer's Disease report 2011-2012.

Bloss et al. (2011). Understanding the Biology of Alzheimer's Disease and Aging Brain. Working memory loss in normal aging.

Britannica encyclopedia on immune theory.

Brion, J.P. *Eur Neurol.* (Oct 1998). 40(3):130-40. (www.ncbi.nlm.gov/pubmed/9748670): Neurofibrillary tangles and Alzheimer's disease.

Bulgarelli, Marco (2013). Periyar River Pollution. © 2013 MarcoBulgarelliJoomla! Is Free Software released under the GNU General Public License.

Casserly, I., Topol, E. Lancet (2004). Convergence of atherosclerosis and Alzheimer's disease: inflammation, cholesterol, and misfolded proteins. Cross Ref, PubMed, CAS, Web of Science®.

Corder, Sandy (2008). Yahoo Contributor Network December 16.

Chun, W. and Johnson, G.V. (2007). The Role of Tau Phosphorylation Front Biosci. 12:733–56. doi: 10.2741/2097. PMD.

Dallas, Mary Elizebeth (August 6, 2012). Working with Diacetyle may risk of proteins clumping.Nlm.nih.gov.

DeKosky, Steven (Jan 28, 2014). Link between pesticide DDT and Alzheimer's Disease.

Dobson, C.B., Itzhaki, R.F. (1999). "Herpes Simplex virus type 1 and Alzheimer's Disease. *Neurobiol. Aging* 20 (4): 457-65.

Eur Neurol. 1998 Oct, 40 (3): 130-40: The neurons are the main processing cells in the brain.

Francis, P.T., Palmer, A.M., Snape, M., Wilcox, G.K. (1999). The cholinergic hypothesis of Alzheimer's disease: a review of progress. *J.Neurol. Neurosurg. Psychiatr.* 6666(2):137-47, xx.

Games, D. (1995). Alzheimer-type Neuropathology in Transgenic Mice Overexpressing V717F Beta-amyloid Precursor Protein. *Nature.* 373(6514):523–27. doi:10.1038/373523a0author2=Adams D. PMID 7845465.

Garg et al. (2011). "Astrocytes and Blood vessels in Aging and Alzheimer's and Brain aging". Understanding the Biology of Alzheimer's Disease and the Aging. National Institute of Aging.

Ginlio Maria Pasinetti MD. (2009). Type-2 diabetes and Alzheimer's: public release: date 10 April. The Mount Sinai Hospital/Mount Sinai School of Medicine.

Goedert, M., Spillantini, M.G., Crowther, R.A. (1991). Tau Proteins and Neurofibrillary Degeneration. *Brain Pathol.* 1(4):279–86. doi:10.1111/j.1750-3639.1991.tb00671.x. PMID 1669718.

Hardy J. Allsop, D. (1991). 12(10): 383-88: Amyloid deposition as the central event in the aetiology of Alzheimer's disease.

Hemera/Thinkstock 2012. "The Butter Flavorant Diacetyleof chemical Research in Toxicology." American Chemical Society, News release, Aug, 1, 2012.

Heneka, M.T. et al. (2010). Locus ceruleus controls Alzheimer's disease pathology by modulating microglial functions through norepinephrine. *Proc Natl Acad Sci USA*. 107:6058–6063. doi:10.1073/pnas.0909586107 PMID 20231476.

Henrich, R.W. (1990). Concurrent and emergent applications of neuropsychological assessment: Problems of Validity and utility Professional Psychology. *Research and Practice,* 21, 3, 171-76.

Holmes, C. and Cotterell, D. (December 2009). "Role of infection in pathogenesis of AD: Implications for treatment" *CNS Drugs* 23 (12):993-1002.

Iqbal, K. (2005). Tau Pathology in Alzheimer Disease and Other Tauopathies. *Biochim Biophys Acta.* 1739(2–3):198–210. doi:10.1016/j.bbadis.2004.09.008. PMID 15615638.

Israel et al., National Institute of Health; National Institute of Aging 2011-2012 Alzheimer's Disease Progress report.

Itzhaki, R.F., et al. (January 1997). "Herpes Simlex Virus Type 1 in brain and risk of AD" *Lancet.* 349 (9047):241-4 PMD 9014911.

Izhaki, R.F. and Wozniak, M.A. (May 2008). "HSV type 1 in AD: the enemy within. *Alzheimer's Disease* 13 (4): 393-405 PMID 1888487848.

Jacob Roy M.D. et al., The Dementia India Report 2010.

Jeri McBryde. (November 2, 2010). About Alzheimer's: Blood vessel theory as a possible cause of Alzheimer's disease.

——. (November 3, 2010). About Alzheimer's. Alzheimer's disease: Possible cause, the slow virus theory.

John's Hopkins University (May 19, 2000). New Nervous Theory on Allergy Emerging.

José A. Luchsinger MD, MPH, Richard Mayeux MD. (2004). Cardiovascular risk factors and Alzheimer's disease. Taub Institute for Research of Alzheimer's. Curr Atheroscler Rep. 2004 Jul; volume 6, issue (4):261-66. Contact: Alzheimer's Association PR, media@alz.org 312-335-4078 Alzheimer's Association.

Kastenholz, B. et al. (2009). "Plant Metal Chaperones: A Novel Perspective in Dementia Therapy". Amyloid 16 (2): 81-83.

Katherine, J. et al., "Tau accumulation causes Mitchondrial Distribution Deficits in Neurons in a Mouse model of Taupathy and in Human Alzheimer's Disease Brain. *The American Journal of Pathology*. Vol. 179, No. 4, October 2011 AND Understanding the Biology of Alzheimer's Disease and Aging Brain. NIH 2011-2012. Alzheimer's Disease Progress Report, Institute of AGING.

Kitazawa, et al., 2011. (University of California) National Institute of aging. Alzheimer's Progress Report. Understanding the Biology of Alzheimer's Disease and Brain Aging. Chronic Inflammation contributes to neurodegeneration in Alzheimer's Disease.

Koo, E.H. et al. (Feb. 1990). Precursor of amyloid protein in Alzheimer disease undergoes fast anterograde axonal transport. *Proc Natl Acad Sci U S A*. 87(4):1561-1565.

Ksiezak-Reading, H. et al. (1994). "Ultrastructure and biochemical composition of paired helical filaments in corticobasal degeneration" [Ultrastructure and biochemical composition of paired helical filaments in corticobasal degeneration]. *American Journal of Pathology* 145 (6): 1496-508. PMC 1887493. PMID 7992852 reported by National Institute of Health, National Institute of Aging.

Landau, S.M., et al. (Jan. 23, 2012). Association of lifetime cognitive engagement and low B-amyloid deposition. Archives of Neurology. Published online Jan. 23, 2012. Page last updated: February 13, 2013.

Latimer et al., 2011. Understanding the Biology of Alzheimer's disease and Aging Brain; National Institute on Aging 2011-2012 Alzheimer's Progress Report.

Li, Q.X. and Whyte, S. Tanner (1990). Secretion of Alzheimer's disease A-beta amyloid peptide by activated human platelets: University of Melbourne.

Lottit, Ne and Head, E. (2005). Alzheimer Disease and Down syndrome: factors in pathogenesis. *urobiol Aging*. 26 (3):383-89.

Luchisinger, J.A. and Mayeux, R. (2004). Cardiovascular Risk factors and Alzheimer's Disease. *Curr Atheroscler Rep*. July. 6 (4): 261-66.

Mahley, R.W., Weisgraber, K.H. and Huang, Y. (2006). Apolipoprotein E4: A Causative Factor and Therapeutic Target in Neuropathology, Including Alzheimer's Disease. *Proc. Natl.* Academy.sci USA.103 (15):5644-51 (Cited by Wikipedia).

Manuelidis, Elias E. and Laura Manuelidis. "Suggested Links between Different Types of Dementias: Creutzfeldt-Jakob Disease, Alzheimer Disease, and Retroviral CNS Infections." *Alzheimer Disease and Associated Disorders*, 2 (1989): 100-09.

Markesbery, W.R. Oxidative stress Hypothesis in Alzheimer's Disease. Sanders-Bown Center on Aging, Lexington, KY 40536-0230, USA. *Free Radic Biol Med. 1997*, 23(1): 134-47.

McGeer, E.G. and McGeer, P.L. (2010). Neuroinflammation in Alzheimer's disease and mild cognitive impairment: a field in its infancy. *Journal of Alzheimer's Disease.* 19(1):355-61.

McKhann, Guy, David Drachman, Marshall Folstein et al. on Alzheimer's Disease. "Clinical Diagnosis of Alzheimer's Disease." *Neurology,* 34 (1984):939.

Milan, Fiala, Dr. John Ringman, and Dr. Francesco Chiappelli, *Journal of Alzheimer's Disease*, June 10, 2 Department of Internal Medicine and Therapeutics, Geriatric Section, University of Pavia, ASP, IDR Reviewed by William J. Netzer, Ph.D., Fisher Centre for Alzheimer's Research Foundation at The Rockefeller University.

MMRC/BHF Heart Protection Study of antioxidant vitamin supplementation in 20,536 high-risk individuals: a randomized placebo.

Möller, H.J. and Graeber, M.B. (1998). Modern Alzheimer's Disease Concept. *Eur Arch Psychiatry Clin Neurosci.* 248 (3):111-22.

Nistor, M. (2007). Alpha-and Beta-secretase activity as a function of age and beta-amyloid in Down syndrome and normal brain. *Neurobiol aging.* 28(10):1493-1506.

Perry, R.T., Go, R.C., Harrell, L.E. and Acton, R.T. (1995). *Am J Med Genet* 60: 12-8.

Petersen, R.C. et al. (2005). Vitamin E and donepezil for the treatment of mild cognitive impairment. *N. Engl. J. Med* 2005; 352: 2379-88. CrossRef, PubMed, CAS, Web of Science®.

Polvikoski, T. (1995). Apolipoprotein E., Dementia, and Cortical Deposition of Beta-amyloid Protein. *N Engl J Med*. 333(19):1242–47. doi: 10.1056/NEJM199511093331902. PMID 7566000.

Prusiner, Stanley (January 31, 2007). What really causes cow disease? Wsired. Retrieved. Retrieved 2007-01-02.

Pyles, R.B. (2001). The association of Herpes Simplex virus and AD disease; a potential synthesis of genetic and environmental factors (PDF). Herpes 8 (3): 64-8. PMD 11867022.

Ramanan, V.K., et al. (Feb. 19, 2013). APOE and BCHE as modulators of cerebral amyloid deposition: a florbetapir PET genome-wide association study. *Molecular Psychiatry*. Published online.

Richard Barrans Jr., Slow Virus-NEWTON Ask a Scientist at Argonne National Labs! www.newton.dept.anl.gov/askasci/bio99/bio99484.htm.

Sardi, F., Fassina, L., Venturini, L., et al., "Alzheimer's disease, autoimmunity and inflammation. The good the bad and the ugly." Source: Margherita, via Emilia 12, Pavia, Italy. *Autoimmunity Reviews*, Volume 11, Issue 2, December 2011, 149-153.

Seshadri Sudha, M.D., Alexa Beiser, Ph.D., Jacob Selhub, Ph.D., Paul F. (February 14, 2002); *N Engl J Med* 2002; 346:476-483. 10.1056/NEJMoa011613 Plasma Homocysteine as a Risk Factor for Dementia and Alzheimer's Disease.

Sonnen et al. (2011). National Institute of Health; Institute of Aging; Understanding the Biology of Alzheimer's Disease and Aging Brain.

Stampfer, M.J. *J Intern Med*. 2006 (3):211-23.

Stampfer, M.J., Kang, J.H., Chen, J., Cherry, R., Grodstein, F. Effects of moderate alcohol consumption on cognitive function in women. *N Engl J Med* 2005; 352: 245-53.

Strittmatter, W.J. Apolipoprotein E: High-avidity Binding to Beta-amyloid and Increased Frequency of Type 4 Allele in Late-onset Familial Alzheimer Disease. *Proc Natl Acad Sci USA*. 1993; 90(5):1977–81. doi:10.1073/pnas.90.5.1977. PMID 8446617.

Sue, B., Wang, X., Nunomura, A., et al. (December 2008). Öxidative stress signaling in Alzheimer's Disease. *Curr Alzheimer's Res* 5(6):525-32.

Taupin, P. Adult neurogenesis, neuroinflammation and therapeutic potential of adult neural stem cells. *Int J Med Sci* 2008; 5(3): 127-32.

Teixeira, F., et al. "Clinico-pathological correlation in Dementia." *Journal of Psychiatry and Neuroscience*, 20 (1995):276-282.

Tiraboschi, P. et al. (2004). The importance of neuritic plaques and tangles to the development and evalution of AD. *Neurology.* 62(11): 1984-89.

Turner, P.R., O'Connor, K., Tate, W.P., Abraham, W.C. (2003). Roles of Amyloid Precursor Protein and its Fragments in Regulating Neural Activity, Plasticity and Memory. *Prog. Neurobiol.* 70(1): 1-32. doi: 10.1016/S0301-0082(03)00089-3. PMID 12927332.4.

Turner, T.H. et al. (2007). Effects of 42 hour sleep deprivation on component processes of verbal working memory "*Neuropsychology* 21(6):787-795.

Verkhratsky, Alexie. et al. (2011-2012 ADD). Understanding the Biology of Alzheimer's disease and aging brain; National Institute of Aging 2011-2012.

Waring, S.C., Rosenberg, R.N. Genome-wide Association Studies in Alzheimer Disease. *Arch Neurol.* 2008; 65(3):329-34.

Waymire, Jack C. Acetylcholine function: Neuroscience on line University of Texas Medical School at Houston.

Wozniak, M.A., Mee, A.P., Itzhaki, R.F. (January 2009). "Herpes Simple Virus type 1 DNA is located within AD Amyloid Plaques" (1) 131-8. *Pathol.*217. PMID 18973185J.

Yao et al. (2011). Mitochondrial Dysfunction in Alzheimer's Disease. Understanding the Biology of Alzheimer's Disease and Aging Brain. National Institute of Aging.

Zina Kroner, D.O. 2009. *Alternate Medicine Review* Vol. 14, No. 4, 2009. Type 3 diabetes.

3

Pollution

Pollution is a major issue with population growth and environmental quality. Although India knows that population growth may contribute to environmental degradation, the government believes that its effects can be modified by economic growth and modern technology.

Water Pollution

Water is highly polluted due to untreated sewerage. Ganges and Yamuna rivers that are heavily polluted meander through highly-populated areas. Pollution has marred the beauty and sanctity of Taj Mahal. Pure water supply and sanitation are inadequate. Water pollution is described as: Raw sewage running into lake or streams; industrial waste spills contaminating groundwater; radiation spills or nuclear accidents; illegal dumping of substances, or items in bodies of water; biological contamination such as bacteria growth; organic material decay in water supplies. India has to clean all the water ways to protect its people from diseases.

Air Pollution

India is the world's largest consumer of fuel wood, agricultural waste and biomass for energy purposes. Fuel wood, agriculture waste and biomass cake burning release over 165 million tons of combustion products into India's indoor and outdoor air every year. Vehicle emissions are worsened by fuel adulteration and poor fuel combustion efficiencies from traffic congestion and low density of quality, high speed road network per 1000 people. India is the third largest emitter of total carbon. In addition, forest fires, volcanic eruptions, dry soil erosion, and other natural sources; building construction or demolition contaminate air. Health outweighs development.

Physician for social responsibility of USA reported the following on pollutants and stroke. When harmful air pollutants lead to inflammation and artery blockages in the arteries that nourish the brain, they can lead to stroke. Stroke is an important cause of incapacitation and of death. Particulate matter, especially fine particulates (PM2.5), increase the risk of strokes and death from strokes, especially for women. Data from the Women's Health Initiative show that for each increase of 10 $\mu g/m^3$ in the PM2.5 concentration, women faced a 35 per cent increase in the risk of a cerebrovascular event and an 83 per cent increase in the risk of death from a cerebrovascular event.

Although a relatively small portion of all strokes appear to be related to concentration of PM, the fact that nearly 800,000 people in the U.S. have a stroke each year means that even a small percentage results in a significant number of strokes. Studies have also found correlations between sulphur dioxide concentrations and ischemic stroke, carbon monoxide and stroke, and ozone peak concentrations and stroke. Sulphur dioxide is an environmental hazard.

Mercury and Developmental Damage

Mercury is a potent neurotoxin that can severely harm the brain and the developing nervous system. Human exposure to mercury occurs as a result of air pollution from natural sources such as volcanoes, but also from man-made sources like coal-fired power plants, cement kilns and industrial boilers. These sources emit mercury into the atmosphere, where it remains until it is carried back to the earth by the rain. When mercury enters lakes and streams, bacteria convert it to methyl mercury, a chemical form that accumulates in the tissues of fish and animals and moves up the food chain. Humans are exposed primarily through fish consumption, with large tuna, swordfish, king mackerel, and tilefish having the high levels of methyl mercury. When pregnant women eat foods contaminated with methyl mercury, they expose their developing babies to lead.

Solid Waste

Trash and garbage are a common sight in urban and rural areas of India. It is a major source of pollution. Indian cities alone generate more than 100 million tons of solid waste a year. Public places and sidewalks are polluted with filth and litter; rivers and canals act as garbage dumps. Solid waste is a mammoth problem to manage unless government in each state makes it a point to conduct scientific research to solve the problem before the solid waste produce unforeseen diseases. In Chennai, the Cooum and Adayar Rivers are highly polluted. Mosquitoes are in abundance in these places that generate unforeseen diseases. Garbage and contaminated water can produce pathogens like Salmonella, E. coli and disease known and unknown to man. These pathogens make people very sick. Virus unknown to man is spreading in cities. The *Times of India*, Chennai, July 2, 2013 carries the caption "Undiagnosed infectious fever puzzles city Docs." "In the past few weeks, many hospitals have been seeing several cases of 'undiagnosed fever' with patients showing symptoms similar to those of malaria, dengue, Japanese encephalitis and typhoid. However the physicians are in a spot as the infectious disease test results turn out to be negative making it difficult for them to understand the ailment and prescribe medications."

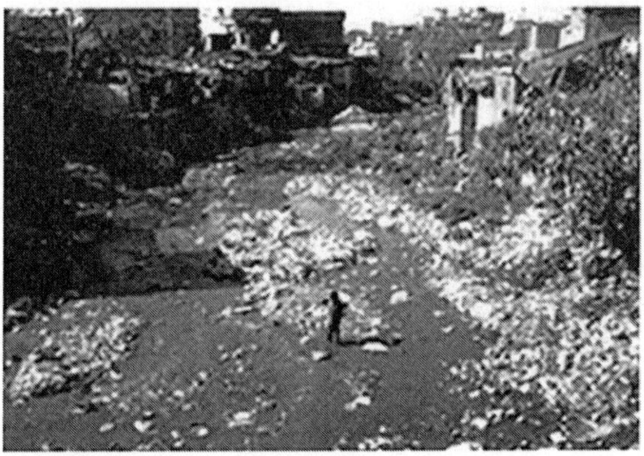

Solid waste

Public pressure is driving industry and government to innovate faster than they would like to find solutions.

Noise Pollution

The Supreme Court of India gave a significant verdict on noise pollution in 2005. Unnecessary honking of vehicles makes for a high decibel level of noise in cities. The use of loudspeakers for political purposes and for sermons by temples and mosques, churches make noise pollution in residential areas worse. In January 2010, Government of India published norms of permissible noise levels in urban and rural areas. Recently, high ranking retired army officers in Coonoor, a hill station in Tamil Nadu, complained about the dinning sounds emanating from a temple that disturbed their peaceful retired life and their sleep. The retired people of hill stations, enjoy reading a book with a cup of tea beside them out in the garden occasionally taking a peek at the overpowering scenic beauty of nature and listening to the birds. They enjoy taking a long walk and ending up in the Coonoor Club for the evening social activities. Ear drum bursting noise is harmful to the human.

Noise pollution is any loud sounds that are either harmful or annoying to humans and animals. Some examples of noise pollution are: airplanes, helicopters and motor vehicles, traffic, rail roads, construction or demolition noise; human activities such as sporting events or festivals like Holi in India. Undisturbed sleep is absolutely necessary for the self-repairing process of the brain. Noise pollution is disruptive to humans' stress levels, may be harmful to unborn babies, and drives animals away, causing nervousness and decreasing their ability to hear prey or predators.

Land Pollution

Land pollution is responsible for damage done to natural habitat of animals, deforestation and damage done to natural resources, and in all, making the communities look ugly. Some examples of land pollution include: litter found on the side of the road; illegal dumping in natural habitats; oil spills that happen inland; damage and debris caused from unsustainable mining and logging practices; radiation spills or nuclear accidents. Land pollution is due to pesticides, fertilizers, in certain areas due to fly ash ponds of thermal power stations, as well as corrosion. Land pollution is also due to poor garbage disposal services in both rural and urban areas of India. Bengaluru that is known as Garden City of India is now called Garbage City.

Greenhouse Gas Emissions or Chemical Pollution

On per capita basis, India emitted about 1.4 tons of carbon dioxide per person in comparison to the United States 17 tons per person and a world average of 5.3 per person.

Thermal Pollution: It is the increase of temperature caused by human activity. Warmer lake water from nearby manufacturing using cool water to cool the plant and then pump it back into the lake; included in thermal pollution is also the increase in temperatures in areas with lots of concrete or vehicles, generally in cities.

Light Pollution: Light pollution is the over illumination of an area that is considered obtrusive. Sources include: large cities; billboards and advertising; night time sporting events and other night time entertainment. Light pollution makes it impossible to see stars, therefore interfering with astronomical observation and personal enjoyment. If it is near residential areas, light has adverse health effects and wastes energy. Light pollution disrupts ecosystems and is dangerous to nocturnal wildlife and plants and trees. Another pollution that is mentioned is visual pollution. Some buildings in front of one's home can mar the view of nature and awful looking structures around one's home can be distressing.

Visual Pollution: It can be caused by other pollution or just by undesirable, unattractive views. It may lower the quality of life in certain areas, or could impact property values and personal enjoyment. Sources of visual pollution include: Power lines; construction areas; billboards and advertising; neglected areas or objects such as polluted vacant fields or abandoned buildings. While visual pollution has few immediate health or environmental effects, what's causing the eyesore can have detrimental effects.

Personal Pollution: Personal pollution is the contamination of one's body and lifestyle with detrimental actions. This may include: Excessive smoking, drinking or drug abuse; emotional or physical abuse; poor living conditions and habits; poor personal attitudes.In some cases, personal pollution may be inflicted by caregivers, while in other cases it is caused by voluntary actions. Taking positive steps in your life can help eliminate this and other sources of pollution so you can lead a more productive, satisfying life. Learn to fight pollution. All these pollutions are interconnected.

Conservation

Ecological issues are an integral part of environmental issues challenging India. It has very dense forests to Mangrove to scrub cover. It has Arabian Sea, Indian Ocean and Bay of Bengal surrounding it; it has high mountain ranges and dense forests that give shelter to tigers, wild elephants and other animals. It is a sanctuary for rare birds and butterflies of varied hues and colors. When one wakes up in the morning to the sounds and cooing of birds, it can be predicted that the day is going to be fruitful. High ranges in southern Western Ghats, was the essence of picturesque beauty. The forests were adorned with majestic trees of oak, sandalwood, rosewood, champak and very many medicinal trees and plants. Magnolia, rare fruit trees and orchids of several varieties living on the trunks of host trees and rare variety of fauna and flora that existed in these forests in the past are extinct. Flora and fauna are endangered today. In olden days, herd of elephants blocked the roads and the leopards crossed the roads. Bisons are a rarity today. The tea and cardamom estates were kept clean in the past, so also the roads but not now. The thick mist that moves mysteriously into the drawing room and the cool breeze with the aromatic air mixed with special scents of flowers from the forests transport one to a world of unparalleled quietness and peace. Forests supply abundance of oxygen for the brain. Champak, magnolia, jasmine and rose flowers contain fragrances that are alluring, medicinal and positively stimulating the brain while the water falls bring pure water for people. The laughing sounds of the waterfalls is lulling and pacifying.

After I lived in USA for forty years I returned to Munnar. It was agonizing to see how people had destroyed the land that epitomized beauty of the wild and the miracle of the earth. Deforestation has been extensive in Kerala and Uttarakhand. These two governments do not respect the key conservation laws in the country including the Indian Wildlife (Protection) Act, 1972, Forest (Conservation) Act, 1980 and Environmental (Protection) Act, 1986. The high ranges forest is replaced with banana trees, tapioca and jack fruit trees. "Ozone that is vital in the atmosphere for filtering sunlight and protecting us from UV is also a killer when it is closer to the ground causing respiratory problems and damaging crops.—Scientists predicted that the conversion of rainforests to plantation—to meet increasing demand for food or fuel—could increase the level of pollutants and Ozone to harmful levels." ("Good up high, bad nearby", Climate chemistry and the tropics: by University of Cambridge. News letter dated 27/06/14).

Munnar Town was known as "Little London (UK)" during the time of Britishers who owned and managed the tea estates, spanning 250 square miles. Now Munnar Town looks like a shanty town all dilapidated and musky with road side tiny tea shops with garbage piled up and litter strewn all around. These are rat-infested garbage piles. The town is dirty and filthy. What kinds of pathogens lurk in these piles of dirt and filth? No one knows.

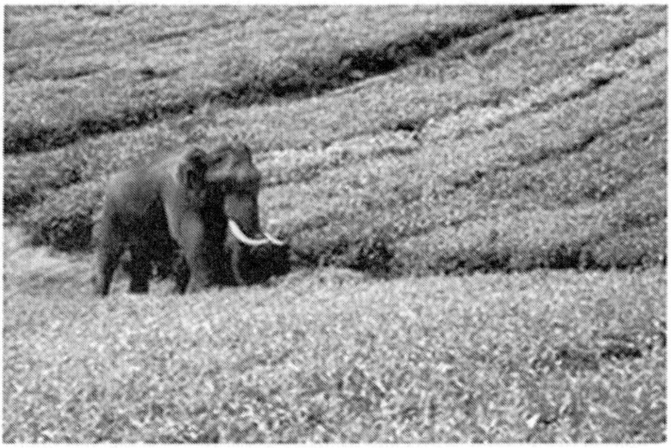

High Ranges, Munnar. Tea estate and rogue elephant

Most of the homes in southern India burn sandalwood sticks in the morning and place jasmine and toses to propitiate gods, whom they worship. Most women in South India adorn their hair with these flowers as well, not only as adornment, but it denotes religious significance. The aroma exuding from the fragrant flowers make people vibrant, happy and divinely peaceful. These flowers have medicinal properties as well. Deforestation has eradicated many medicinal plants that have been used in Ayurvedic medicines. Deforestation produces greenhouse effect on our planet. Forests removed carbon dioxide (CO_2) from the atmosphere, prior to deforestation.

Beautiful things and aromatic scents make people happy and relaxed. (Refer to five senses in prevention chapter.) This is one of the reasons why people go to parks, on excursions or vacations to scenic beautiful places to relax. All the senses are vital to enjoy life. Filthy surroundings can only make people depressed and physically sick. All the senses have centers in the brain and these senses have to be activated to appreciate nature and life. All sensations are coded in the brain and information is stored in long-term memory. Senses have strong connections to emotional memory. Tranquil environmental scenes such as the sea or a beach, can positively affect the human brain function, according to research published. Nature scenes help brain to function (Pa.Press.net, 15.09.2001).

Study of smell on Alzheimer's: Cardiff University, Professor Tim Jacob, School of Biosciences is studying the olfactory function in humans: How and why do we smell? The olfactory bulb is one of the structures of the limbic system and a very ancient part of the brain. The information captured by the sense of smell goes from the olfactory bulb to other structures of the limbic system. The limbic system is also concerned with translating sensory data from the neo-cortex (the thinking brain) into motivational forces for behavior. In any case, good smell is relaxing and bad smell is revolting to the senses.

Man displaced the animals and now the elephants are encroaching upon the lands inhabited by people. The depletion of global forests and their degradation are causes for concern as they involve not only the loss of forest areas, but also the ultimate quality of the forests. If this trend is unchecked, the implications on the world would be cataclysmal. Not only would the existence of all forest types be threatened, but the capability of these forests to perform their various roles and functions in perpetuity would also be seriously undermined. Hence, the need to address the decline in global forest areas and its degradation through enhancing forest cover is immediate.

The following poem is written by Talin M. Kathare, an eight-year-old, student of Vale's Billabong, an International School in Chennai, India.

"Respect Nature"

Nature has no limits; Nature doesn't have to be green,
Neither an elephant, nor a tiger nor a tree,
Nature has been given everything, for them to be!
Even if humans fight or if monkeys act as donkeys,
Nature loves all of us as one
How can we survive with all our techno devices?
Nature is so important, Nature is so sweet
So just do your best to respect nature and she will do the rest.

This poem was illustrated with pictures of a plant, a tree, a tiger and an elephant.

To quote Mahatma Gandhi, on Kerala, India:

"Kerala, the sunny, lush, green State lies between the Lakshadweep Sea and the Western Ghats mountains in southern peninsular India. It is nourished by 44 rivers and a chain of backwaters. Its physiography and its culture are unique. The verdant forests, pristine rivulets and golden beaches are nature's priceless gifts to Kerala."

The earth has enough
for everyone's needs
but not enough
for some people's greed.

The Dementia Report of 2010 on Alzheimer's reported that Kerala state has the highest rate of incidence of Alzheimer's. The reasons are yet to be studied at length.

Kerala in South India is known worldwide as 'God's own country' because of the breath-taking scenic and prosperous nature. The backwaters are unique in the world, a network of lakes, canals and deltas of forty-four rivers flow into the Arabian Sea. The backwaters of Kerala are a self-supporting eco-system teeming with aquatic life. The largest backwater stretch in Kerala is the Vembanad Lake, which flows through three districts and opens out into the sea at the Kochi Port. Mahatma Gandhi will be shocked to see the present Kerala.

Eloor is an island of 14.21 km formed between two distributaries of river Periyar and is the largest industrial belt in Kerala with 247 chemical industries. As a result of its heavy industries, it is heavily polluted and is rated as one of the toxic hotspots of the world. It houses the one and only DDT factory which releases continuous offensive strong odor. DDT is as organic pollutant. The air is toxic, so also the water in the lakes and rivers. There is hardly any drinking water in Eloor. The Periyar River carries the contaminated acidic water through lakes and into the Arabian Sea and on its way destroys the agricultural land and the aquatic life. The soil and water are contaminated with metals like zinc, lead, chromium, and cadmium which is similar to zinc and mercury. Cadmium is extremely poisonous. The air in Eloor is thick with acid mists, ammonia and chlorine. Persistent Organic pollutants (POPs) directly threaten public health and the surrounding environment. "There is an overwhelming increase in most types of systemic diseases; the organs affected are the neoplasm blood and the blood forming organs, the endocrine, nutritional and metabolic systems, mental and behavioral problems due to the affection of the nervous system and many more. Every organ in the body seems affected. Safe drinking water is not available for majority of people in Eloor." Illegal sand mining leads to ecological niche and habitat of various biotic forms. According to Marco Bulgarelli (2013)—Chalakudy River in Kerala is equally polluted. It is reported that Chalakudy also has high rate of incidence of Alzheimer's."

Pesticide Exposure Risk: DDT Linked to Heightened Alzheimer's Risk

The pesticide DDT is banned in the U.S. because of its toxic effects on wildlife and potential to harm human health, may raise the risk for Alzheimer's disease, according to the first study linking the chemical to the brain-ravaging illness. People with Alzheimer's disease had about four times the level of DDT. By-product in their blood compared with those who didn't have the dementia, according to the research published yesterday in the journal *Neurology*. People exposed to DDT are at higher risk of AD, particularly if they carry a particular apolipoprotein E (APOE) genotype.

Steven DeKosky, professor of Neurology at the University of Virginia, recommended that the researchers should look at the environmental factors for AD and suggested that researchers may conduct studies on pesticides. "We are exploring a lot of ways that the environment may predispose us to or protect us from neurodegenerative diseases later in life. This is a new clue that we will chase down" (JAMA *Neurology*; Jan. 28, 2014).

The main types of pollution are: water, air, soil, thermal, radioactive, noise, and light pollution.

REFERENCES

DeKosky, Steven. Jan. 28 (2014). JAMA Neurology; DDT and Alzheimer's Disease.

Marco, Bulgarelli (2013). Periyar River Pollution.

Nicole, Ostrow Jan. 28 (2014) 10:31: Bloomburg news. Pesticide DDT Linked to Increased Alzheimer's risk.

Pa.Press.net.15.09.(2001). Nature scenes help brain to function.

Physician for social responsibility of USA (36)201: PM2.5 and stroke.

Times of India, Chennai; July 2 (2013): "Undiagnosed infectious fever puzzles city Docs".

University of Cambridge newsletter dated 27.06.(2014). Climate chemistry and the tropics.

4

Stages of Progression of Alzheimer's and Techniques for Evaluations

The loss of grey matter in Alzheimer's disease is found first in memory-related areas of the brain known as the hippocampus and the entorhinal cortex. This is followed by areas that affect 'cognitive' functions, namely the temporal, frontal and parietal lobes and midbrain. Midbrain controls movements. The increasing difficulties with memory, cognition, thinking, conceptualization, behavior and motor problems seen in Alzheimer's disease are a reflection of this progressive damage to the different lobes and other parts of the brain.

Depletion of Neurotransmitters

Neurons communicate with each other through an electrochemical process. The chemical is known as neuro-transmitters. In Alzheimer's, the neurotransmitter called Acetylcholine is generally found to be depleted. Many of the medications used to slow down the symptoms of Alzheimer's disease work by enhancing the levels of this neurotransmitter. Acetylcholine is involved in many aspects of brain functions. Acetylcholine is vital in the functioning of memory, learning, problem-solving, judgment, decision-making and other aspects of cognition and as well as some aspects of behavior. (Wikipedia encyclopedia and Kendra Cherry About.education). *Note*: Gasotransmitters are gaseous molecules synthesized in the body. They include nitric oxide, hydrogen sulfide, and carbon monoxide.

Other neurotransmitters can also be affected in people with Alzheimer's disease. For example, memory problems have been linked to the loss of neurons containing glutamate. In addition, behavioral problems in people with Alzheimer's disease have been linked to loss of neurons containing dopamine. Depressive symptoms can be due to the loss of neurons containing norepinephrine and sleep problems can be due to the loss of neurons containing serotonin. The brain has several different chemicals. The major chemicals, the neurotransmitters, are serotonin, dopamine and norepinephrine (Wikipedia encyclopedia) and (what is neurotransmitter by Kendra Cherry, About.education).

ALZHEIMER'S DISEASE

Diagnostic and statistical manual of mental disorders IVth edition gives diagnostic criteria for Alzheimer's.

Disorders included are: Cognitive deficits, language and communication difficulties and forms of aphasia, apraxia and agnosia, personality and behavior.

Neuropsychological tests are administered to test areas of language difficulties.

1. Visual agnosia where the person has difficulty in recognizing objects, faces and words. 2. Auditory agnosia which involves the inability to recognize sounds. 3. Somatosensory agnosia where the person has difficulty to perceiving objects through tactile stimulation (Joseph G. Chusid; 16th edition). Agnosia is usually considered to be caused by disturbances in the association function of the cerebral cortex. These difficulties cause a person to be dysfunctional in activities of daily living.

Orientation, concentration, comprehension, learning, language, communication and memory are limited in Alzheimer's. Personality changes and behavior changes are other features of AD.

Researchers work on three stages, five stages and seven stages of Alzheimer's.

NEW CRITERIA FOR DIAGNOSIS OF AD 2012 SET BY NIA AND ALZHEIMER'S ORGANIZATION

1. Preclinical AD.
2. MCI (Mild Cognitive Impairment) due to Alzheimer's disease.
3. Dementia due to Alzheimer's disease.

Preclinical AD

During this stage, individuals have measurable changes in the brain. Cerebrospinal fluid and/or blood (biomarkers) that indicate the earliest signs of disease, but they have not yet developed memory loss. However, no diagnostic criterion is established.

Preclinical Stage

Three stages of Alzheimer's by *Brain Today* was published on April 19, 2011. It refers to the new guidelines, developed by the National Institute of Aging and the National Alzheimer's Association. At this stage there are no clear signs of AD. In the Preclinical Alzheimer's disease, there are no symptoms but there are measurable changes in the brain evidenced by the biomarkers. These include protein levels in the brain, blood and spinal fluid. It is estimated that brain changes occur as many as 20 years before symptoms are evident.

Mild Cognitive Impairment (MCI) Due to Alzheimer's Disease (NIA-2012)

A mild but measurable change in thinking abilities takes place but it does not affect ADLs. Alzheimer's Association and NIA report that 10 per cent to 20 per cent of adults over 65 years of age and older have MCI. This population can manifest symptoms of AD in three to four years. When individuals with MCI develop AD then MCI is actually an early stage of the particular form of dementia, rather than a separate entity. Biomarker testing is recommended in such cases. Biomarkers are changes in the brain, cerebrospinal fluid and/or blood are caused by physiological processes associated with AD. If these factors are present, then a diagnosis of MCI can be made.

Dementia Due to Alzheimer's Disease

Cognitive impairment interferes with an individual's ability to function in daily life and is caused by Alzheimer's disease-related processes. (Alzheimer's Association, 2012a.)

The Progression of Alzheimer's

Alzheimer's disease progressively affects memory, thinking, and behavior. According to the Global Deterioration Scale (Alzheimer's Association, 2012d and NIA), there are seven key stages of Alzheimer's development.

According to *Brain Today* (2011), at this stage AD has underlying pathology consistent with AD. They also will have memory disturbances and other cognitive deficits. It is postulated that this stage is predictive of disease process that will progress toward AD. At this stage the brain is still relatively healthy.

Kronkosky of Charitable Foundation ALZHEIMER'S DISEASE, on May 2012 and NIA note The Progression of AD.

Stage One: No cognitive impairment

- No Cognitive impairment.
- No memory problems evident.

Stage Two: Very mild cognitive impairment

- Memory lapses for familiar words and names.
- Lapses not evident to friends, family, co-workers, or doctors.

Stage Three: Mild cognitive decline

- Friends, family, and co-workers begin to notice deficiencies in memory.
- Problems with memory, retention and concentration.
- Difficulty naming objects or people.
- Decreased performance of daily activities.
- Decline in abilities to plan or organize.

Stage Four: Moderate cognitive decline

- Clear-cut deficiencies in knowledge of recent events.
- Decreased capacity to perform complex tasks such as planning, for thanks giving.
- Dinner or managing finances.
- Demeanor may be subdued or withdrawn.

Stage Five: Moderately severe cognitive decline

- Major gaps in memory and cognitive functioning.
- Need for assistance with daily functions.
- Confusion about location and date.

Stage Six: Severe cognitive decline

- Increased memory deficits.
- Significant personality changes.
- Difficulty recalling personal history.
- Tendency to wander and become lost.
- Impaired ability to execute common actions such as dressing oneself.

Stage Seven

- Very severe cognitive decline.
- Little to no ability to speak.
- Failure to recognize objects and people.
- Loss of voluntary muscle control.
- Assistance required for all daily functions.

  (Fisher Centre and Alzheimer's Disease, Research Brief of May 2012 by Alzheimer's Association. This scale has seven stages).

  Mayo clinic has more or less the same criteria as above.

Alzheimer's Society, England

The progression of Alzheimer's disease (12/2013).

Alzheimer's disease is a progressive illness. This means that the structure and chemistry of the brain become increasingly damaged over time. The person's ability to remember, understand, communicate and reason will gradually decline. Looking at Alzheimer's disease as a series of three stages can be a useful way of understanding the changes that occur over time. But it is important to realize that this view of Alzheimer's can only provide a rough guide to the course of the disease. This is because:

Some symptoms may appear earlier or later than indicated here, or not at all, the stages may overlap—the person may need help with one task, but may be able to manage another activity on his own.

Some symptoms such as walking about, may appear at one stage and then vanish, while others such as memory loss will worsen over time.

The way that a person experiences Alzheimer's disease will depend on many factors, including their physical make-up, their emotional resilience, the medication they take and the support they can rely on.

Early Stage

Alzheimer's disease usually begins gradually with very minor changes in the person's abilities or behavior. At the time, such signs are often mistakenly attributed to stress or bereavement or, in older people, to the normal process of ageing. It is often only when looking back that we realize that these signs were probably the beginnings of dementia.

"Loss of memory for recent events is a common early sign. Someone with Alzheimer's may:

- forget about recent conversations or events
- repeat themselves
- become slower at grasping new ideas
- lose the thread of what is being said
- sometimes become confused
- show poor judgment, or find it harder to make decisions
- lose interest in other people or activities
- develop a readiness to blame others for taking mislaid items
- unwilling to try out new things or adapt to change."

If you are caring for someone with Alzheimer's disease, there's a lot you can do in the early stages to help the person you are caring for maintain their independence. It may be tempting to do things for them, but they are more likely to retain their sense of self-worth if they are given the chance to do things for themselves, with support if necessary (see factsheet staying involved and active).

The person may also become anxious and agitated. They may experience distress over their failure to manage tasks and may need some reassurance. If this is the case, try to talk to them, and give them as much emotional support as you can.

Middle Stage

As Alzheimer's disease progresses, the changes become more marked. The person will need more support to help them manage their day-to-day living. They may need frequent reminders or help to eat, wash, dress and use the toilet. They are likely to become increasingly forgetful—particularly of names—and may sometimes repeat the same question or phrase over and over because of the decline in their memory for recent events. They may also fail to recognize people or confuse them with others.

Some people at this stage become very easily upset, angry or aggressive—perhaps because they are feeling frustrated—or they may lose their confidence and become very clingy. Other symptoms may include:

- becoming confused about where they are, or walking off and becoming lost (disorientation for place).
- becoming muddled about time and getting up at night because they are mixing up night and day (disorientation for time and confusion between day and night).
- putting themselves or others at risk through their forgetfulness—for example, by not lighting the gas on the cooker (cognitive disturbance).
- behaving in ways that may seem unusual such as going outside in their nightclothes (inappropriate behavior).
- difficulty with perception, and in some cases having hallucinations (reality testing difficulties).

For more information about these symptoms and how to deal with them, see factsheets on unusual behavior; moving and walking about and sight, perception and hallucinations in dementia.

Late Stage

At this stage, the person with Alzheimer's will need even more help and will gradually become totally dependent on others for nursing care. Loss of memory may become very pronounced, with the person unable to recognize familiar objects or surroundings or even those closest to them, although there may be sudden flashes of recognition.

The person may also become increasingly frail. They may start to shuffle or walk unsteadily, eventually becoming confined to bed or a wheelchair. Other symptoms may include:

- difficulty in eating and sometimes swallowing
- considerable weight loss—although some people eat too much and put on weight
- incontinence—losing control of their bladder and sometimes their bowels as well
- gradual loss of speech, though they may repeat a few words or cry out from time to time.

The person may become restless, sometimes seeming to be searching for someone or something. They may become distressed or aggressive—especially if they feel threatened in some way. Angry outbursts may occur during close personal care, usually because the person does not understand what is happening. Those caring for the person should try not to take this personally; the person is not being aggressive deliberately.

Although the person may seem to have little understanding of speech, and may not recognize those around them, they may still respond to affection and to being talked to in a calm soothing voice. They may also enjoy scents, music, or stroking a pet.

On average, people with Alzheimer's disease live for eight to ten years after their symptoms begin. Life expectancy does, however, vary considerably depending on how old the person is. For example, people diagnosed in their 60s and early 70s can expect to live for around seven to ten years, whereas someone diagnosed in their 90s will, on average, live for about three years. The length of time that someone with dementia can expect to live for also depends on whether they were diagnosed early on or later in the disease.

The Three Stages of Alzheimer's Disease Proposed by the 2011 Criteria and Guidelines (NIA)

The three stages of Alzheimer's disease proposed by the 2011 criteria and guidelines are: (1) preclinical Alzheimer's disease, (2) mild cognitive impairment (MCI) due to Alzheimer's disease, and (3) dementia due to Alzheimer's disease. Those who have very mild symptoms but can still perform everyday tasks would be described as having MCI due to Alzheimer's. Individuals who have more pronounced symptoms that interfere with carrying out everyday tasks would be said to have dementia due to Alzheimer's disease.

Preclinical Alzheimer's Disease

An individual who does not yet have outward symptoms of Alzheimer's but does have some of the early brain changes of Alzheimer's (as detected by brain imaging and other biomarker tests) would be said to have preclinical Alzheimer's disease.

"Individuals have measurable changes in the brain. Cerebrospinal fluid and/or blood (biomarkers) that indicate the earliest signs of disease, but they have not yet developed noticeable symptoms such as memory loss. This preclinical or pre-symptomatic stage reflects current thinking that Alzheimer's related brain changes may begin 20 years or more before symptoms occur. Although the 2011 criteria and guidelines identify preclinical disease as a stage of Alzheimer's, they do not establish diagnostic criteria that doctors can use now. Thus, additional research is needed before this stage of Alzheimer's can be identified."

Mild Cognitive Impairment (MCI) Due to Alzheimer's Disease

Those who have very mild symptoms but can still perform everyday tasks would be described as having MCI due to Alzheimer's. Individuals who have more pronounced symptoms that interfere with carrying out everyday tasks would be said to have dementia due to Alzheimer's disease. Individuals with MCI have mild but measurable changes in thinking abilities that are noticeable to the person affected, to family members and others. MCI does not affect the individual's ability to carry out everyday activities. Cognitive decline is more likely among individuals whose MCI involves memory problems than among those whose MCI does not involve memory problems. When an individual with MCI goes on to develop dementia, many scientists believe that the MCI is actually an early stage of the particular form of dementia, rather than a separate condition.

'Disease modifying' treatment will be most effective when administered during the preclinical and MCI stages of the disease. Biomarker tests are vital to identify the individuals who will be receiving disease modifying treatment. Which biomarker or a combination of biomarkers will be most effective for diagnosis of Alzheimer's is yet to be established.

2014 Facts and Figures: New criteria set by (NIA) National Institute of Aging and Alzheimer's Association.

1. They identify three stages of Alzheimer's disease, with the first occurring before symptoms such as development of memory loss. In contrast, for Alzheimer's disease to be diagnosed using the 1984 criteria, memory loss and a decline in thinking abilities must have occurred.
2. They incorporate biomarker tests. A biomarker is a biological factor that can be measured to indicate the presence or absence of disease, or the risk of developing a disease. Levels of certain proteins in fluid (for example, levels of beta and tau in the cerebrospinal fluid and blood) are among several factors being studied as possible biomarkers for Alzheimer's.

Current research by Sara Westwood at Kings College, London reports that "this study has identified longitudinal blood-based biomarkers of brain pathology and cognitive decline. Proteins that can predict how much amyloid will be present in the brain 12 years later on have also been identified." Researchers report that 'A new type of Brain scan' may detect Alzheimer's early, using no radiation and at less cost than other techniques. Doctors at the University of Pennsylvania's Perelman School of Medicine have developed a form of Magnetic Resonance Imaging, or MRI, that detects brain changes that signal Alzheimer's disease. The doctors have developed a modification to the technique called Arterial Spin Labeling or ASL-MRI. Preliminary studies show that this may be a useful way to diagnose probable early dementia.

Medical Imaging to Detect AD with a Camera by University Michigan: It is actually the PET (Positron emission tomography). It can be used to identify AD.

"PET scanning is a way to look at the brain in people who are living and dealing with their disease," says Norman Foster, M.D., the U-M neurologist leading the research team. "The PET machine looks very much like an MRI or CT scanner, but it's different because it can show not just what the brain looks like inside the head, but how active different parts of the brain are and how they are reacting to the disease." This brain activity or lack of it is what matters in Alzheimer's disease, adds Foster, who directs the Cognitive Disorders Clinic at the U-M Geriatrics Center and is a professor in the U-M Department of Neurology and associate director of the Michigan Alzheimer's Disease Research Center.

"Though the causes are mostly unknown, save for a suspected genetic link in some cases, the effects are all too apparent. Patients who start out with absentmindedness and mild memory loss worsen to become restless, moody, anxious, and confused, with increasing memory loss. In the final stages, patients often lose the ability to talk to others or care for themselves."

G8 Summit UK in 2012-13: David Cameron, Prime Minister, allocated funds for Brain Scans for some NHS patients with complicated symptoms.

The degeneration of a small, wishbone-shaped structure deep inside the brain may provide the earliest clues to future cognitive decline, long before healthy older people exhibit clinical symptoms of memory loss or dementia, a study by researchers with the UC Davis Alzheimer's Disease Center has found. This study is led by Evan Fletcher. The key importance of this finding is that it suggests that white matter tract measures may prove to be promising candidate biomarkers for predicting incipient cognitive decline among cognitively normal individuals in a clinical setting, possibly more so than gray matter measures," he said. "Brain circuitry Loss may be an early sign of Cognitive Decline" (Sept. 9, 2013).

REFERENCES

Acta Neuropathol. 1991; 81(3):261-8: Alzheimer's disease affects limbic nuclei of the thalamus.

Alzheimer's Association, and NIA (2012). Global Deterioration Scale

Alzheimer's Association, May (2012). Fisher Centre and Alzheimer's Disease

Alzheimer' Society, December (2013). Three stages of the Progression of Alzheimer's Disease.

Brain Today April 19 (2011). Three stages of Alzheimer's.

Chusid, Joseph G., 16th edition: Correlative *Neuroanatomy & Functional Neurology,* Lange Medical Publications, Los Altos, California 94022.

Evan Fletcher, Sep. 9, (2013). Brain Circuitry Loss may be an Early Sign of Cognitive Decline.

Facts and Figures (2014). New criteria set by (NIA) National Institute of Aging and Alzheimer's Association.

Kendara Cherry : Neurotransmitters. About.education

Mayo clinic: Alzheimer's stages: How the disease progresses by Mayo Clinic staff.

Norman Foster, M.D. Sep. 9 (2013). PET measures different parts of the brain and how they are reacting to the disease. (University of Michigan).

University of Pennsylvania. Nov. 16 (2011). ASL-MRI Arterial spin Labeling.

Wikipedia free encyclopedia. List of neurotransmitters.

5

Lobes of the Brain and Their Functions

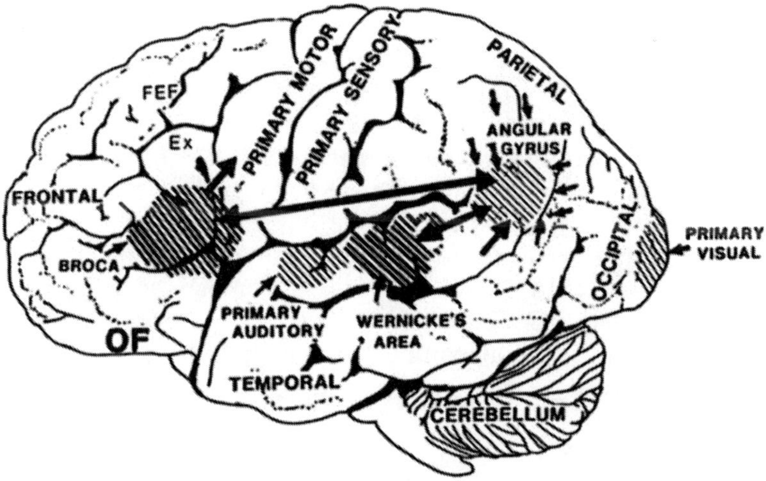

Source: Wikipedia encyclopedia.

NEURON

The Neuron is also known as nerve cell. All sensations, movements, thoughts, memories and feeling are the result of signals that pass through neurons. Neurons when they die cannot be replaced like other cells. On the other hand, data published in November 1998 by University of Washington show that in one area of the brain, of the Hippocampus new neurons can grow in adult humans (Faculty of Washington, November 1998).

Neuron has three parts:

(a) Cell body (soma) contains the nucleus.

(b) Dendrites branches out from the cell body and receive messages from other nerve cells. Dendrites bring electrical signals to the cell body. The cell body of a neuron frequently gives rise to multiple dendrites.

(c) Axon is an extension that arises from the cell body. Signals then pass from the dendrites through the cell body and may travel away from the cell body down an axon to another neuron, a muscle cell or cells in some other organ. Axons carry messages from one cell to another in the cortex. Synapse is the place where a signal passes from the neuron to another cell. When the signal reaches the end of the axon, it stimulates tiny sacs. These sacs release chemicals known as neurotransmitters into the synapse. The point of contact of one neuron with another is known as a Synapse. The neurotransmitters cross the synapse and attach to receptors on the neighboring cell. These receptors can change the properties of the receiving cell. If the receiving cell is also a neuron, the signal can continue the transmission to the next cell. Some brain cells have more than 15,000 synapses. In humans, neurogenesis largely ceases during adulthood, but for two brain areas, the hippocampus and olfactory bulb.

Some Key Neurotransmitters at Work

Neurotransmitters are categorized into four groups: Acetylcholine, Monoamines, Amino acids and Peptides.

Acetylcholine is called an excitatory neurotransmitter because it generally makes cells more excitable. It governs muscle contractions and causes glands to secrete hormones. In Alzheimer's, there is deficiency of Acetylcholine. Deficiencies lead to memory disturbances.

GABA (gamma-aminobutyric acid) is called an inhibitory neurotransmitter because it tends to make cells less excitable. It helps control muscle activity and is an important part of the visual system.

Monoamines are: Epinephrine, Norepinephrine, Dopamine and Serotonin.

Monoamines are produced by several system of neuron in the Brain. Monoaminergic neurons serve to modulate the function of widespread regions throughout the brain. They serve as volume controls that increase or decrease the activities of particular functions.

Serotonin is an inhibitory neurotransmitter that constricts blood vessels and brings on sleep. It is also involved in regulation of temperature, eating, and wakefulness and regulation of pain.

Dopamine is an inhibitory neurotransmitter involved in attention and learning; mood and the control of complex movements. The loss of dopamine activity in some parts of the brain leads to the muscular rigidity of Parkinson's in the brain.

Epinephrine and Norepinephrine are also known as adrenaline and noradrenalin. Epinephrine is a hormone produced in adrenal medulla. Norepinephrine is a transmitter substance in the brain. Noradrenergic neurons examine the mechanism that regulates the release and synthesis of the neurotransmitter noradrenaline or norepinephrine. It plays an important role in response to stress and the development of resistance to stress as well as psychological states. (Kendra Cherry about education and Wikipedia the free encyclopedia of Neurotransmitter.)

BRAIN

Anatomically, the brain is divided into Telencephalon and Diencephalon. The Telencephalon include Cerebral Cortex, Basal Ganglia and the Limbic system. The Diencephalon consists of a complex collection of nuclei lying symmetrically on either side of the midline. Diencephalon includes the Thalamus, Hypothalamus, Epithalamus and Subthalamus.

Cerebral Cortex

The cerebral cortex is divided into right and left hemisphere. The brain has several lobes with specific functions in terms of cognition, language, visuomotor functions, remembering, problem solving, thinking and feeling.

Right Hemisphere Versus Left Brain

The left hemisphere of the brain is considered dominant due to its superior language abilities, analytic and sequential abilities. It has the linguistic abilities including verbal intelligence and memories. This is inclusive of talking, reading, speech, communication, verbal intelligence and memories. Right brain is responsible for information processing in the area of mathematics, grammar, logic, analytic reasoning and interpretation of details.

Right hemisphere is not linguistically based but deals with non-verbal material in the likes of perception of people's faces and details, geometrical patterns, interpretation of the body language of a person. It gives meaning to social cues. It is responsible for creativity, insight and intuitive reasoning. It guides visual spatial processing thereby rendering understanding of material at hand. However, these two hemispheres work in unison. The Corpus Callosum is the structure deep in the brain that connects the right and left hemispheres of the cerebrum, coordinating the functions of the two halves.

American Speech and Language-Hearing Association note the symptoms of right hemisphere brain damage as follows: Speech pathologists work with Aphasic patients.

1. **Attention:** Difficulty to concentrate for more than a few minutes at a time.
2. **Left-side neglect:** Individual no longer realizes the left side of the body. Individual affected may not eat food that is on the left of the plate. While reading the patient will read from the middle of the page, neglecting the left side.
3. **Memory:** Problems remembering information such as street names or important dates, and learning new information easily.
4. **Orientation:** Difficulty recalling the date, time, or place. The individual may also be disoriented to self, meaning that he/she cannot correctly recall personal information such as birth date, age, or family names.

5. **Organization:** Trouble telling a story in order, giving directions, or maintaining a topic during conversations.
6. **Problem-solving:** Difficulty in responding appropriately to common events such as a car breakdown or overflowing sink. Leaving the individual unsupervised may be dangerous in such cases, as he or she could cause injury to himself or herself, or others.
7. **Reasoning:** Difficulty in interpreting abstract language such as metaphors, or responding to humor appropriately.

Social communication (pragmatics): Problems understanding non-verbal cues and following the rules of communication, (e.g. saying inappropriate things, not using facial expressions, talking at the wrong time (American Speech-Language-Hearing Association 2013) (Left Brain vs Right Brain by Kendra Cherry, About.com education).

Cerebral Hemisphere is divided into four lobes: Frontal, Parietal, Temporal and Occipital Lobes.

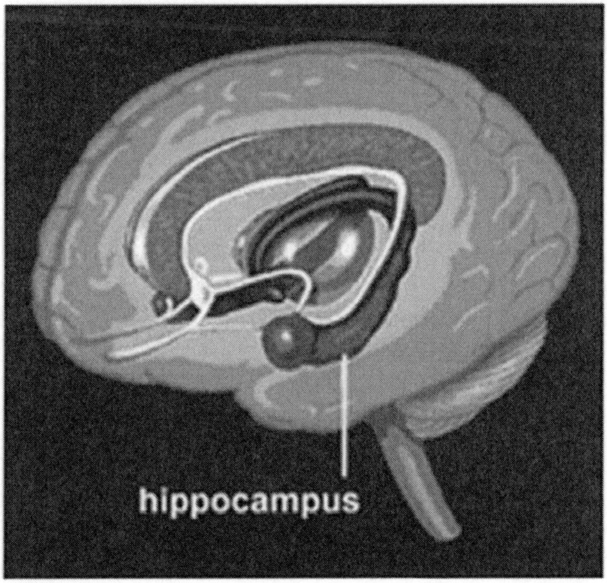

Source: Wikipedia

FRONTAL LOBE

The frontal lobe (FL) contains most of the dopamine sensitive neurons in the cerebral cortex. The dopamine system is associated with reward, attention, concentration, long term memory, short-term memory tasks, planning and motivation. Dopamine tends to limit and select sensory information arriving from Thalamus to the forebrain. Frontal lobe monitors expressive language. It has the executive abilities; it plans, organizes, is goal oriented, positive and productive. FL maintains social decorum, empathy and altruism. It controls voluntary muscles used for running, dancing, and all kinds of movements. It also contributes to Spatial Orientation and position of the body in space.

SYMPTOMS OF FRONTOTEMPORAL DEMENTIA

Northern University Cognitive Neurology and Alzheimer's disease states that this is a type of dementia called "Frontotemporal dementia" which typically affects patients at a very early age. The cell damage caused by frontotemporal dementia leads to tissue shrinkage and reduced function in the brain's frontal and temporal lobes, which control planning and judgment; emotions, speaking and understanding speech; and certain types of movement.

They show impairments in social skills, inappropriate or bizarre social behavior, like doing sit-ups in a public restroom, being overly familiar with strangers and so on. They manifest "loosening" of normal social restraints; for example using obscene language or making inappropriate sexual remarks. Social skills show ineffective human interactions to inappropriate social behaviors. Perseveration, confabulation, and lack of control over emotions are noted. Their thinking can be illogical and accusatory. They generally show lack of judgment and personal space.

FL damage can result in a range of behaviors such as swearing, undressing and urinating in public, eating and drinking non-food items. (Cultural factors to be considered.) Other features of frontal lobe syndromes include reduced activity, particularly a diminution of spontaneous activity, lack of drive, inability to plan ahead, and lack of concern. Sometimes associated with this are bouts of restless, aimless uncoordinated behavior. Affect may be disturbed with apathy, emotional blunting. The patient may show an indifference to the world around him. In contrast, on other occasions, euphoria and disinhibition are described. The euphoria is not that of a manic condition, but having an empty quality to it. The disinhibition can lead to marked abnormalities of behavior, sometimes associated with outbursts of irritability and aggression. When frontal lobe degenerates, all the above positive functions will deteriorate depending on the status of the progression of AD. The deterioration takes place gradually from mild, to moderate to severe. Deterioration will take place in the areas of cognition, thinking, communication, memory, executive functions, emotions, moods, social behaviors and personality. According to a report from NIMH this could be due to a gene variant.

What is Frontotemporal Dementia? By Alzheimer's Society, England

Frontotemporal dementia is caused when nerve cells in the frontal and/or temporal lobes of the brain die and the pathways that connect them change. There is also some loss of important chemical messengers. Over time, the brain tissue in the frontal and temporal lobes shrinks.

As frontotemporal dementia is a less common form of dementia, many people (including some health professionals) may not have heard of it.

Symptoms

In frontotemporal dementia, a variety of symptoms are caused by damage to different areas of the frontal and temporal lobes. Based on these symptoms and the lobes that are affected, a person may have one of three types of frontotemporal dementia:

- behavioral variant frontotemporal dementia;
- progressive non-fluent aphasia; and
- semantic dementia.

As with most forms of dementia, the initial symptoms can be very subtle, but they slowly get worse as the disease progresses over several years.

Behavioral Variant Frontotemporal Dementia

This form is diagnosed in about two-thirds of people with frontotemporal dementia. During the early stages, changes are seen in the person's personality and behavior.

A person with behavioral variant frontotemporal dementia may:

- lose their inhibitions—behave in socially inappropriate ways and act in an impulsive or rash manner; this could include making tactless or inappropriate comments about someone's appearance.
- lose interest in people and things—lose motivation but (unlike someone with depression) they are not sad.
- lose sympathy or empathy—become less responsive to the needs of others and show less social interest or personal warmth; this can make the person appear selfish and unfeeling.
- show repetitive, compulsive or ritualised behaviors—this can include repeated use of phrases or gestures, hoarding and obsessions with timekeeping.
- crave sweet or fatty foods, lose table etiquette, or binge on 'junk' foods, alcohol or cigarettes.

Language Variants of Frontotemporal Dementia

In both of the language forms of frontotemporal dementia, other aspects of mental function (memory, visuospatial skills, planning and organising) tend to be well preserved in the early stages.

Later Stages

In the later stages of all forms of frontotemporal dementia, damage to the brain becomes more widespread. Symptoms are often then similar to those of the later stages of Alzheimer's disease.

For details of Alzheimer's Society services in your area, visit alzheimers.org.uk/localinfo

For information about a wide range of dementia-related topics, visit alzheimers.org.uk/factsheets

When Frontal Lobe is Damaged the Following Features may be Evident

Impairment of higher cortical functions like concentration, thinking, creative thinking, abstraction, and conceptualization may be evident. Other features are memory difficulties, lack of spontaneity, lack of ability to communicate. Frontal lobe damage may show symptom of Aphasia, Apraxia, Agnosia, and Acalculia. Any one of these higher order functions will be deteriorated.

Plaques and tangles begin to form in brain areas involved in learning, memory, thinking and planning. As the disease advances, the region that deals with memory, thinking and planning develop more plaques and tangles than were present in early stages. In an advanced stage most of the cortex of the AD is seriously damaged. The brain shrinks dramatically due to widespread cell death. Individuals lose their ability to communicate, to recognize family and loved ones and to care for themselves. In some people loss of smell and/or taste can occur. Inability to express language may be found if Broca's area is affected.

The following characteristics of the frontal lobe syndrome will be helpful to Neuropsychologists. Thimble (1990) also gives guidelines for Neuropsychological Evaluation and Assessment.

Clinical Characteristics of the Three Principal Frontal Lobe Syndromes: Michael H. Thimble, F.R.C.P., FRC Psych, 1990 conducted seminars on frontal lobe syndrome and frontotemporal syndrome and orbitofrontal syndrome in 1990.

ORBITOFRONTAL SYNDROME

Originally called Dysexecutive syndrome, it is being looked into and believe that it is not a syndrome. Falls into cognitive, emotional and behavioral.

Cognitive

- Short attention span—may manifest symtoms of ADHD
- Poor working memory
- Poor short-term memory
- Difficulty in planning and reasoning
- Environmental dependence syndrome
- Poor abstraction

Emotional

- Difficulty in inhibiting emotions, anger, excitement, sadness, etc.
- Depression, possibly due to above.
- Occasionally, difficulty in understanding others' points of view, leading to anger and frustration.

Behavioral

- Utilization behavior
- Perseveration behavior
- Inappropriate aggression
- Inappropriate sexual behavior
- Inappropriate humor and telling of pointless and boring stories (Witzelsucht).

Source: Wikipedia free encyclopedia

MEDIAL FRONTAL SYNDROME (AKINETIC)

Paucity of spontaneous movement and gesture; sparse verbal output, apathy, slowness, disinhibition lower extremity weakness, loss of sensation and incontinence. Frontal lobe is a fascinating area to study and thus there are many books written on it. (Other References: Frontal Lobe Biology Regina Bailey about.com and Frontal Lobe-Wikipedia, the free encyclopedia.)

TEMPORAL LOBE

The temporal lobe is located anterior to the occipital lobe and inferior to the frontal lobe and parietal lobe. Temporal lobe is one of the regions in the cerebral cortex and the structures of limbic system inclusive of olfactory cortex, amygdala and the hippocampus. The temporal lobe's main functions are the processing and analysis of auditory information. Temporal lobe's overall functions are auditory perception, memory, speech, and language comprehension, emotional response, visual perception and categorization of objects.

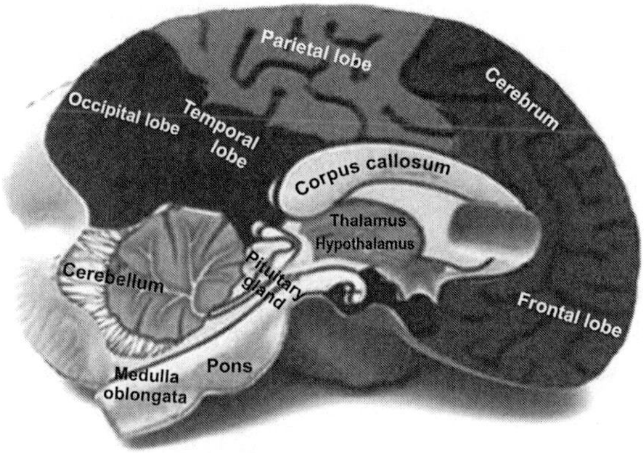

Source: Wikipedia encyclopedia

Temperament is regulated by temporal lobe since visual and auditory functions impact on personality and behavior. The temporal lobe is essential for episodic memory or memory for events. Memory for events will have to be consolidated and encoded, so that events can be retrieved.

Medial TL is responsible for explicit memory which is divided into semantic and episodic memory. Amygdala, brainstem and hippocampus are critical for Long-Term memory. The temporal lobe is involved in the retention of visual memories, processing sensory input, comprehending language, storing new memories, emotions and deriving meaning. The left lobe is involved with, verbal memory like names, verbal features and so on, but the right lobe is involved with visual memory like faces, pictures, places, etc.

The following are the basic functions of the temporal lobe:

1. **Speech** is governed by the left temporal lobe of the brain. This lobe contains the language zone, the Wernicke's

area, which is a part of the brain that is responsible for controlling the mental processing necessary for speech. It controls the processes involved in comprehension and verbal memory.

2. **Memory** is located in the temporal lobe. It stores the essential components of memory that one can recall consciously and describe. These memories can be anything like facts, events, people and places. It plays an important role in retrieving information stored in the brain. It is an important function of temporal lobe.
3. **Reading comprehension and retention:** It Entirely depends on the temporal lobe. It processes the sounds and written words into meaningful information. The temporal lobe allows you to remember what you read and stores the information for you to recollect later.
4. **Emotional responses:** The amygdala, located deep within the temporal lobes plays an important role in processing memory of emotional responses. It enhances mood stability. The deflection in the activity of this lobe can cause fluctuating or unpredictable moods and behavior. The temporal lobe is also concerned with the expression of fear. The temporal lobe, specially the amygdala, processes information related to fear. This applies to expressions of fear felt by others, as well as self-felt fear. Researchers say that the temporal lobe may be stimulated during spiritual or religious experiences. Individuals with temporal lobe epilepsy appear to be highly sensitive to extraordinary experiences.
5. **Auditory responses:** One section in the temporal lobe known as the primary auditory cortex is responsible for receiving and interpreting information that is transmitted through the auditory responses. It responds to different sound frequencies and also helps in determining the location of a particular sound.
6. **Visual process:** The most advanced types of visual memory are processed and interpreted by the lower

portions of the temporal lobe. It is responsible for feelings of conviction and insight.

7. **Olfactory functions:** Olfactory lobe which is responsible for identification and recognition of olfactory information is situated in the lower surface of the temporal lobe (Amruta Deshpande, 3/15/2010). Robert S. Wilson, Julie A. Schneider, Steven E. Arnold, Yuxiao Tang, Patricia A. Boyle, and David A. Bennett. *Arch Gen Psychiatry*. 2007; 64:802-08.

Temporal lobe houses hippocampus and amygdala which regulate memory. The temporal lobes are involved in primary auditory perception and house the primary auditory cortex. The areas related to vision in the temporal lobe offer interpretation to the meaning of visual stimuli to establish object recognition. Damage to temporal lobe can produce disturbances in auditory and visual perceptions, disturbances of language, comprehension and speech. Damage to the temporal lobes, and parts of the frontal lobes, means that while certain objects might be recognized there is little or no ability to process new information and remember it later. Because there are different types of memory each is affected differently according to the severity of damage.

A person with frontotemporal lobes degeneration may be able to speak but sentences may come out disorganized and meaningless. Damage to this area may result in alexia, apraxia and anomia. The most common symptom of inferior temporal lobe damage is visual agnosia. The individual will have difficulties to read, write, and remember the names of objects. Personality changes may occur and the individual may become humorless and may manifest extreme religious perspectives. Individual may have difficulties to recognize and appreciate music; will have difficulties to recognize shape; in interpreting emotions of others and in some cases facial recognition will be impaired. Other observed difficulties are: difficulty in recognizing faces named as prosopagnosia (Benton, A.L., 1980), short-term memory loss, persistent talking, and increased aggressive behavior.

LIMBIC SYSTEM

Limbic system is comprised of amygdala, hippocampus, hypothalamus, thalamus, regions of the limbic cortex and the septal area. These structures form connections between the limbic system, hippocampus and the cortex. The hippocampus is important in memory and learning while the limbic system is central in the control of emotional responses. [The Temporal Lobe and Limbic system by Pierre Gloor (Amazon.com). Squire, LR; Stark, CE; Clark, RE (2004). Other references Temporal Lobe-Wikipedia encyclopedia and Temporal Lobe—The Brain Made simple.com]

HIPPOCAMPUS

Hippocampus stores short term memory related to events that are currently taking place. It processes new memories for long-term storage. The long term storage is the memory of past events which is broken down into how to do things (procedural memory) and language associated memory (declarative which is further divided into semantic and episodic memory). Hippocampus is closely associated with cerebral cortex. Hippocampus plays an important role in the consolidation of information from short term memory (STM) and long term memory (LTM) and spatial navigation. Hippocampus functions are: auditory perception, memory, speech, emotional responses and visual perception.

In ADIs, the hippocampus is one of the first regions of the brain to suffer damage. This produces memory problems and disorientation. Damage to the hippocampus can result from lack of oxygen. People with extensive hippocampus damage may experience amnesia—the inability to learn and retain new memories. Age-related decrease in memory can be caused by Hippocampus deterioration. Limbic system plays a role in the formation and storage of memories associated with emotional event. Emotions and memory are intertwined. Intense emotional events that arouse love, fear and Anger/hatred, laughter are easily embedded (etched) in memory. PTSD is due to experience of intense emotions of anger, fear, anxiety, depression and other emotions. Vietnam veterans who suffer from PTSD suffer from these features. Amygdala is involved in the modulation of memory consolidation as found in mental illness and PTSD. It is easier to erase a bad memory than the emotion behind the bad memory.

Limbic system transfers emotional information into memory. The main location for this transfer is hippocampus. Hippocampus is necessary to make new memories. If hippocampus is damaged, then the person has to live in the past. Early symptoms noted in AD is due to changes in cognition, (intellectual aspects) specifically memory. Cognition and memory rate of deterioration will vary from person to person. If hippocampus is damaged, STM and LTM will be impaired. However, they can learn new skills (procedural memory); may have implicit memory for experiences (Di Gennaro et. al., *Journal of Neurological Sciences*, 27, 129-33. DOI: 10.1007/ s10072).

AD affects the hippocampus first and severely before other parts of the cortex and thus will have difficulties to have new memories. For example, patient could have just given his spouse a cup of coffee and still may ask "is Tom here although he may be standing in front of the patient". "Who visited today?"

Patient who talked to her aunt who visited her and shortly after aunt's departure, the patient may ask "Did she come"? The hippocampus can be damaged through oxygen deprivation or hypoxia. Hippocampus seems to be involved in severe mental illnesses like schizophrenia and severe depression. In these cases, the hippocampus has evidently shrunk.

Age-related conditions such as Alzheimer's disease for which hippocampus disruption is one of the earliest signs (Hampel, et al., 2008) have a severe impact on many types of cognition, but even normal aging is associated with a gradual decline in some types of memory, including episodic memory and working memory. Because the hippocampus is thought to play a central role in memory, there has been considerable interest in the possibility that age-related declines could be caused by hippocampus deterioration (Harrison, P.J. 2004). Some early studies reported substantial loss of neurons in the hippocampus of elderly people, but later studies using more precise techniques found only minimal difference. Similarly, some MRI studies have reported shrinkage of the hippocampus in dementia, Alzheimer's Type.

AMYGDALA

Amygdala regulates emotions, hormonal secretions, memory and autonomic responses associated with fear. It signals the cortex of motivationally significant stimuli such as those related to reward, fear, and social functioning. Amygdala and hippocampus play important roles in memory. It chooses what memories to be stored and where depends on intensity of emotion and event. Amygdala is also involved in the memory consolidation. Greater emotional arousal following the learning of the event enhances a person's retention of that event.

Studies show relevance of amygdala to shyness, hyperactivity, social phobia and borderline personality disorder. In Bipolar disorders, the volume of amygdala is considerably lower and also the volume of hippocampus. The neuropsychological correlates of amygdala activity are: sexual orientation; social interaction; aggression; fear; alcoholism; binge drinking and hemispheric specialization. When in AD amygdala is severely damaged, emotional instability occurs. It is quite common for episodes of paranoia, temper outbursts, and bouts of anxiety to occur due to the damage. In the area of cognition and memory rarely deterioration will vary from person to person.

When the amygdala is damaged in humans, they lose their sensitivity to stimuli associated with strong emotions. For example, Adolphs, Russell, and Tranel (1999) found that a patient with "complete, bilateral damage restricted to the amygdala" was able to tell when a face was sad or happy, but he had lost his ability to discriminate between different levels of emotional arousal. He could not tell a slightly sad face from a very angry face: they all just looked "unhappy" to him. He had the same problem with happy expressions. He could not tell the difference between a face that showed very mild happiness and one that expressed great joy. He showed Impaired Judgments of Sadness but not Happiness Following Bilateral Amygdala Damage (Ralph Adolphs and Daniel Tranel, 1999). To summarize,

(Shira knafo) amygdala is significantly and consistently affected by Aβ (Beta amyloid peptide) both in patients with AD and in mouse models of this disease. Therefore, this region is a central participant in the pathology of AD (Unger et al., 1991) and its damage may be the structural substrate to the frequent emotional, psychological, and memory disturbances seen in this devastating disorder. One finding is that psychopaths have less activation in the amygdala. Study conducted by University of Chicago. (Other references: Amygdala-Wikipedia encyclopedia; Amygdala, Regina Bailey about.com)

PONS

Pons is a motor relay center. Injury to pons can result in motor deficits to paralysis depending on the areas and intensity. Brain stem of which pons is the upper part has three main functions:

1. Is a transit station back and forth from cerebrum to the cerebellum.
2. The brain stem serves as the origin for the cranial nerves except the olfactory nerve and optic nerve.
3. Influence on ANS (Autonomic Nervous System): Consciousness in the form of alertness, motivation, sleep wake cycle. Pons may play an important role in REM (rapid eye movement) cycle of sleep and arousal. This is why brain stem injury is said to be a life threatening injury.

The Basal Ganglia

Basal Ganglia is connected to limbic system. Basal ganglia is responsible for repetitive behavior, reward experience, and focused attention. The caudate begins just behind the frontal lobe and curves back to occipital lobe. Then it sends its messages to frontal lobe. It tells one what to do under certain circumstances. Basal ganglia is in control of movement like in Parkinson—rigidity, poor balance, tremors, weakness and difficulty with initiating movement. Some anatomists believe that amygdala which is a component of limbic system is a part of basal ganglia given its location in the brain.

Caudate Nucleus

"We conclude that the caudate nucleus contributes to behavior through the excitation of correct action schemas and the selection of appropriate sub-goals based on an evaluation of action-outcomes; both processes fundamental to successful goal-directed action. This is in contrast to the Putamen, which appears to sub-serve cognitive functions more limited to stimulus-response, or habit, learning" (The media and the Amygdala, John sexton 26 April 2013).

The Cingulate Gyrus

This provides a pathway from the thalamus to hippocampus providing focused attention to emotionally charged events and memories to smells and tastes. It is an integral part of the limbic system which is involved with emotion formation and processing (1) learning (2) and memory (Kozlovskiy, S.A.; Vartanov A.V. et al. (2012): The Cingulate and Human Memory Processes). An important part of the limbic system, the cingulate gyrus helps regulate emotions and pain. The cingulate gyrus is thought to directly drive the body's conscious response to unpleasant experiences. In addition, it is involved in fear and the prediction (and avoidance) of negative consequences and can help orient the body away from negative stimuli. Learning to avoid negative consequences is an important feature of memory.

THE THALAMUS

The thalamus controls sensory perception and regulation of motor functions. The thalamus receives sensory information and relays it to the cerebral cortex. The cerebral cortex also sends information to the thalamus which then transmits this information to other parts of the brain and brain stem. All sensory input to the brain is connected to nerve cell clusters of the thalamus. Thalamus acts as a two-way relay station, sorting, processing and directing signals from the spinal cord and mid-brain structures to the cerebrum and conversely, from the cerebrum down the spinal cord to the nervous system. It regulates synaptic transmissions during resting states.

> The thalamus translates neural impulses from various receptors to the cerebral cortex, where they are experienced as the appropriate sensations of touch, pain or temperature during the waking state, and it regulates synaptic transmissions, i.e. incoming impulses during resting states. (*Encyclopedia Britannica*)

The thalamus also plays an important role in regulating states of sleep and wakefulness. The thalamus plays a major role in regulating arousal, the level of awareness, and activity. Damage to the thalamus can lead to permanent coma. Thalamus is affected by Alzheimer's. "Severe changes were confined to only a few limbic nuclei. These changes were found in all cases of severe Alzheimer's that the authors studied. It is assumed that these changes considerably hamper the transport of information through limbic circuits" (*Acta Neuropathol*, 1991). Alzheimer's disease affects limbic nuclei of the thalamus (Reference: Thalamus-Educational Portal).

HYPOTHALAMUS

Hypothalamus controls vital survival behaviors and activities such as eating, drinking, temperature regulation, sleep, emotional behavior, circadian rhythm and sex activity. The central nervous system (CNS) and endocrine system are controlled by the hypothalamus. It controls the pituitary gland by secreting hormones, which gives the hypothalamus a great deal of control over many body functions. Hypothalamus monitors numerous bodily functions such as blood pressure, body weight, appetite and including emotions and normal functioning of the body. Hypothalamus is connected with many parts of the central nervous system, including the brain stem, reticular formation, autonomic zones, the limbic forebrain particularly amygdala, septum, diagonal band of Broca, olfactory bulbs and the central cortex.

The hypothalamus is involved in several functions of the body including: autonomic function control; endocrine function control, releases 8 major hormones by the pituitary gland; homeostasis; motor function control; food and water intake regulation i.e. hunger and thirst; sleep-wake cycle regulation; and mediation of emotional responses (Wikipedia, free encyclopedia and regina bailey about.com).

In addition to regulating the release of pituitary hormones, the hypothalamus also influences caloric intake and weight regulation, establishing a stable "set point" for individual weight gain. The hypothalamus also regulates body heat in response to variations in external temperature, determines wakefulness and sleep and regulates fluid intake and sensation of thirst. Injuries or diseases affecting the hypothalamus may produce symptoms of pituitary dysfunction or diabetes insipidus (*Encyclopedia Britannica*; amygdala, regina bailey about.com).

PARIETAL LOBE

The parietal lobe (PL) is located in the middle section of the brain and is associated with processing tactile sensory information such as pressure, touch and pain. A portion of the brain known as the somatosensory cortex is located in this lobe and is essential to the processing of the body's senses. It is associated with cognition including calculating, location and speed of objects, movement, orientation, recognition and speech. Damage to the parietal lobe can result in problems with verbal memory, an impaired ability to control eye gaze and problems with language.

Parietal lobe is the centre for visual spatial abilities, and manipulation of objects in space. Parietal lobe integrates different senses that allow for understanding a single concept. Individuals with damage to left parietal lobe (LPL) is likely to show right parietal left (RPL) confusion, difficulty with writing and math, left right orientation and touch sensation. In addition, PL lesion can produce aphasia (language disorder) and agnosia (inability to perceive objects normally). Damage to RPL can result in neglecting part of the body in space. Individual will show difficulty in assembling objects (apraxia) and drawing. Individual may deny deficits. This can lead to impairment of many self-care skills, such as dressing, washing, cooking; which are vital to daily activities and management of important aspects for survival. PL integrates somasthetic stimuli for recognition and recall of form, texture and weight.

Bi-lateral damage (large lesions to both sides) can cause "Balint's Syndrome," a visual attention and motor syndrome. This is characterized by the inability to voluntarily control the gaze (ocular apraxia), inability to integrate components of a visual scene (simultanagnosia), and the inability to accurately reach for an object with visual guidance (optic ataxia) (Westmoreland et al., 1994). Special deficits (primarily to memory and personality) can occur if there is damage to the area between the parietal and temporal lobes. Left parietal-temporal lesions can affect verbal memory and the ability to recall strings of digits (Warrington and Weiskrantz, 1977). The right parietal-temporal lobe is concerned with non-verbal memory. Right parietal-temporal lesions can produce significant changes in personality. Some common tests for parietal lobe function are: Kimura Box Test (1977) (apraxia) and the Two-Point Discrimination Test (somatosensory).

Lesion of the anterior PL can cause difficulty in recognizing objects by touch. PL stability is necessary for awareness of position of the body in space. Bilateral damage can produce visual difficulties like reaching for objects, visual attention and motor abilities. Damage to the areas between temporal and parietal lobes can produce memory deficits and personality changes. Parietal lobe receives input from number of senses, visual, auditory and vestibular and tactile (blakemore and Frith, 2005; Penfield, W., and Rasmussen, T., 1950). Macdonald Critchley (1953) stated that AD ultimately affects all parts of the brain but people are affected differently as the condition progresses. PLs have an important role to integrate all the senses. As AD advances the above-mentioned features of the lobes will deteriorate. Non-dominant PL receives information from occipital lobe and gives a picture of the world. Damage will result in an inability to recognize faces, surroundings and objects. For instance father could recognize the voice of the daughter but when she appeared before him he could not recognize her (additional reference: Wikipedia encyclopedia and Hippocampus functions by Dr. Ananya Mandal, News editorial, October 16, 2014).

OCCIPITAL LOBE

Occipital lobe contains primary visual cortex. This lobe is responsible for descriptions of the local orientation, spatial frequency and color properties. Although specific functions are attributed to each lobe, most activities require coordination of multiple areas in both hemispheres—right and left hemispheres. Occipital lobe is essential to visual process, but parts of the parietal, temporal and frontal lobes on both sides also process complex visual stimuli. Occipital lobe is involved in processing information from the eyes but occipital lobe interprets what is seen. If damage to occipital lobe does occur, it may lead to an inability to recognize objects. This coupled with degenerative processes in other parts of the brain could explain why the purposes of every day useful objects are not perceived for what they are for example; how to use a bath room, how to dress with the familiar clothes, how to mail a letter while in the post office and so on.

If one occipital lobe is damaged, the result can be homonymous hemianopsia vision loss from similarly positioned "field cuts" in each eye. Occipital lesions can cause visual hallucinations. Lesions in the parietal-temporal-occipital association area are associated with color agnosia, movement agnosia, and agraphia. Damage to the primary visual cortex, which is located on the surface of the posterior occipital lobe, can cause blindness due to the holes in the visual map on the surface of the visual cortex that resulted from the lesions (Kandel, E., Schwartz, J., and Jessell, T., 1991) (additional reference occipital lobes—regina bailey about.com and occipital lobe—Wikipedia, the free encyclopedia).

CEREBELLUM

Functions of cerebellum are:

1. Coordination of voluntary movements, balance, equilibrium.
2. Some memory for reflex motor acts.

Problems if Impaired

Difficulty with coordination of movements; difficulty to walk or even loss of abilities to walk; difficulty to reach out to take objects; tremors, dizziness (vertigo); slurred speech; inability to make rapid movements.

The cerebellum is comprised of small lobes and receives information from the balance system of the inner ear, sensory nerves, and the auditory and visual systems. It is involved in the coordination of motor movements as well as basic facets of memory and learning.

REFERENCES

Lobes of the Brain, their functions and functions affected by Alzheimer's *Neuropathol.* 1991; 81(3):261-68. Alzheimer's disease affects limbic nuclei of the thalamus.

1. Anatomy of the brain and The Four Lobes. By Kendra Cherry, Center for Neuroskills;
2. Brain structures and their functions,seredip.brynmaur.edu/
3. Brain-Wikipedia, the free encyclopedia;
4. Parts of the Brain and their functions-MD-Health.com.

Adolphs Ralph and Daniel Tranel.Amygdala: *Wikipedia and Journal of Cognitive Science,* 1999, 16-3, pp. 453-62.

Albert, M.L. (1973). *Neurology*, 23, 658-64: A Simple Test of visual neglect.

Alzheimer's society 12.2013: What is Fronto Temporal Dementia?

American Speech-Language-Hearing Association (2013). Right Brain Damage.

Occipital Lobe

Benton on Prosopagnosia: The neuropsychology of face recognition. *Am, Psychol.* 35: 176-86.

Blakemore and Frith (2005). *The Learning Brain*. Blackwell Publishing.

Encyclopedia Britannica: Thalamus.

Frontal Lobe syndromes: Clinical charactgeristic of the three Principal Frontal Lobe Syndromes.

Gauthier, L., Dehaut, F., Joanette, Y. (1989). The Bells Test: A quantitative and qualitative test for visual neglect. *Int J Clin Neuropsychol*, 11, 49-54.

Hampel, H., Bürger, K., Teipel, S.J., Bokde, A.L., Zetterberg, H., Blennow, K. (2008). *Alzheimer's and Dementia*, 4 (1): 38-48. "Core candidate neurochemical and imaging biomarkers of Alzheimer's disease".

Kendal, cherry: About.com: What is Neuron?

Kenneth, M. Heilman and Edward Valenstein. Oxford University Press second edition (1985). *Clinical Neuropsychology*.

Kimura, D. (1977). Acquisition of motor skill after left hemisphere damage. *Brain*, 100:527-42.

Knafo Shira : Amygdala in Alzheimer's Disease. Intechopen.com/book/ the amygdala-a-discrete-multitaking-manager/amygdala-in-alzheimer's disease.

Kolb, Bryan and Ian et al. *Fundamentals of Human Neuropsycholgy*. W.H. Freeman and Company, New York.

Kosslyn Smith (2007). Temporal Lobe.

Macdonald Critchley, December 1 (1953). Parietal Lobes. Macmillan USA.

Michael H. Thimble, September 1990. Psychopathology of Frontal Lobe Syndromes. Clinical Characteristics of the Three Principal Frontal Lobe Syndromes. Neuron: Wikipedia and https/faculty. Washington.edu/chudler/cells.html. November (1998).

Northern University Feinberg of Medicine. Cognitive Neurology and Alzheimer's Disease Center (1990): Frontotemporal Dementia .

Regina Bailey. Hypothalamus About.com and Wikipedia.

——. Occipital Lobes About.com and Wikipedia.

Schulman, K.I. *Int J Geriatr Psychiatry*. (2000) Jun, 15, (6):548-61.

Shulman, K.I., Gold, D.P., Cohen, C.A., Zucchero, C.A. Cloak drawing and dementia in the community: a longitudinal Study. *Int J Geriatr Psychiatry*. 1993; 8: 487-96.

Squire, L.R., Stark, C.E., Clark, R.E. (2004). The medial temporal, lobe. *Annual Review of Neuroscience*, 27: 279-306.

Stuss, D.T., Gow, C.A., and Hetherington, C. (1992). 'No longer gage': Frontal lobe dysfunction and emotional changes. *Journal of Consulting and Clinical Psychology*, 60(3), 349-59.

Warrington and Weiskrantz (1977). The right parietal-temporal lobe is concerned with non-verbal memory.

6

Neuropsychological Assessment

Neuropsychological assessment is carried out in order to gauge the extent of neurological dysfunctions incurred due to a neurological disorder and in this case due to dementia of Alzheimer's type. Currently, there are highly sophisticated instruments in the form of CT, MRI, PET, SPECT to assess the extent of brain damage. The neurologists, neurosurgeons and other referral sources want recommendations regarding the functional abilities, varied treatments options that may help the patient to function optimally, with or without assistance. The neuropsychologist makes recommendations for rehabilitation, habilitation and cognitive stimulation therapy (CST). In order to diagnose dementia, researchers have to use several diagnostic devices in the nature of medical imaging.

Computed Tomography of the Brain (CT or CAT)

CT scans of the brain can provide more detailed information about brain tissue and brain structures than standard X-rays of the head; thus providing more information related to injuries and/or diseases of the brain.

Single-photon Emission Computed Tomography (SPECT)

SPECT imaging is different from the anatomical MRI or CT scans. SPECT measures blood flow and activity patterns. It looks at how the brain works. It is similar to positron emission tomography (PET) scans, which looks at glucose metabolism. When using SPECT imaging, physicians look for three things: Areas of the brain that work well; areas of the brain that are low in activity and areas of the brain that are high in activity.

Magnetic Resonance Imaging (MRI)

Magnetic resonance imaging (MRI) of the brain and brain stem uses magnetic fields and radio waves to produce high quality two or three-dimensional images of brain structures without use of ionizing radiation (X-rays) or radioactive tracers.

Positron Emission Tomography (PET)

PET scan is an imaging test that uses a radioactive substance (called a tracer) to look for disease or injury in the brain. Unlike magnetic resonance imaging (MRI) and computed tomography (CT) scans, which reveal the structure of the brain, a PET scan shows how the brain and its tissues are working. The alternative names are: brain nuclear medicine scan; brain positron emission tomography.

PET/CT Scans and Brain Disorders

Diagnosis of a brain disorder is based on symptoms, medical history, physical examination, risk factors, and clinical tests. Diagnostic procedures may be needed to confirm a diagnosis and imaging tests such as computed tomography (CT), magnetic resonance imaging (MRI), angiography, positron emission tomography (PET), and Doppler Ultrasonography are commonly used to diagnose neurologic disorders.

The selection of neuropsychological tests depends on referral questions and clinical judgment of the patient. The patient in question has his/her own identity and characteristics. They may have different levels of education, ethnicity, different types of occupations, socio-economic status and so on which may affect the test results. Henrich, R.W. in 1990 used a term known as Ecological Validity. The study of the patient has to be anchored within the patient's background.

The evaluations may start with the study of all the documents available on the patient, collateral history and clinical observations. Choice of tests depends on referral questions. Neuropsychologists have several tests with them to address the referral questions and questions raised during clinical interview. Over the years several new tests have been standardized.

Alzheimer's patients go through several stages of progression and one has to keep in mind the fact that different functions deteriorate at different rate. In some cases, progression of Alzheimer's may be very slow and in some unpredictable. Memory deficits are noted early on and so also learning deficits. There are varied opinions on learning abilities of AD patients. Naming objects, remembering names of people whom they met recently may indicate early signs of AD. However, one has to interview the ADIs closely to differentiate between early AD and every day forgetfulness. It is very important to evaluate the purpose of claiming to be AD. Some of them referred to me were not AD. The so-called ADs were looking for certification to get disability benefits.

The diagnoses confirming AD may start with hesitancy to talk and likely to show perplexity and likely to mutter, "What is that, oh I cannot find the word". They may show slight confusion when asked personal questions, may even be undecided. They may have confusion between words. Verbal fluency will be limited. Thus, language and communication will be limited. These features will limit the social life of the person. 'Less the speech, the less the social life.' The language associated speech and communication thus will diminish over time. Brain stimulation also gets diminished. ADIs will manifest difficulties gradually in all areas of functioning. One has to give special attention to differentiate between the speech and communication between very old people and people who suffer from Alzheimer's. Older people will be slow to communicate and may not complete sentences but memory is still satisfactory.

The neuropsychologists may choose tests to measure: attention, concentration, intelligence, memory, language and communication, visuo spatial abilities, dementia-specific abilities, and battery assessing multiple neuropsychological functions and if need be administer personality tests.

Wechsler Adult Intelligence Test is routinely administered to assess various aspects of intelligence, including attention and concentration, thought process, problem-solving abilities, verbal abilities and concept formation, general knowledge and so on. Wechsler series have included Wechsler Test of Adult reading. This test may be administered to ADIs to evaluate abilities to read, comprehend, and remember. This test also may indicate other aspects of brain impairment. Premorbid intelligence can be estimated by "hold tests" which are resistant to cognitive damage. It is debatable in the case of Alzheimer's patients.

Concentration

The clinical model of concentration is described as the sustained focus of cognitive resources on information while filtering or ignoring extraneous information. To me concentration is the absolute shutting out of extraneous stimuli while I am on a topic to study which may involve learning and memory. Digit Span and Arithmetic subtests of WAIS-111 and 1V are good to assess attention and concentration when formally testing a patient. Mental control and digit span of WMS-1V are predictive of attention and concentration. Trail making test A and B are popularly used by neuropsychologists to measure concentration abilities. Digit modalities test also is used to assess concentration.

MEMORY

Over the years experimental and cognitive psychologists have been researching on memory. Cognitive psychology has researched several types of memory. With short-term memory (STM) or (Working memory, or primary memory, these are computer language) information is accessible immediately. In order to store information it has to be rehearsed or else it will be lost. Long-term memory is when memories are stored between a few minutes to several hours or years. LTM is divided into declarative and implicit memory. Declarative is divided into episodic and semantic memory.

Storing Implicit and Explicit Memories: Explicit Memory or declarative is a type of long-term memory requiring conscious thought. It refers to facts and experiences that one can consciously know and declare. Implicit memory is a major form of long-term memory that does not require conscious thought. It involves learning an action while the individual does not know or declare what the individual knows. Examples are cycling, swimming (Wikipedia Encyclopedia).

Episodic memory which stores chronologically events in one's life is impaired in ADIs. Linguistic comprehension deteriorates in AD. AD patients have greater difficulties in the area of communication than speech and language. Episodic memory is autobiographical; a record of personal experiences. Where were you when Edward Kennedy was shot? What do you remember about Tsunami in India? Do you remember where you were when your sister got married? Emotionally charged scenes are easily recalled or retrieved. Highly charged emotional events are easily recorded. All sensory events are recalled if an individual focus on such events.

Interference Theory

In retroactive inhibition, new learning interferes with the retention of old memories. Old memories are changed by new ones, may be even so much that the original one is completely lost. In proactive inhibition, old memories interferes with the retention of new learning. Both are important for human learning.

Then there is the false memory where one can construct and reconstruct memories of events. This is reported in court cases. Ego centric bias: The person puts oneself in the best possible light and so on. In AD patients, both primary and secondary memories are impaired.

Executive functions are an all-encompassing term for various cognitive processes and sub-processes. The executive functions include: problem-solving, planning, organizational skills, selective attention, inhibitory control and some aspects of short-terms memory (Wikipedia). Wikipedia lists a whole gamut of tests to evaluate executive functions. Some of them are: behavioral assessment of dysexecutive syndrome (BAD), Delis-Kaplan executive function which includes Halstead category test; PASAT; stroop test; and many more. To measure visuospatial area Wikipedia mentions Clock Test; Hooper Visual organization (VOT) and Rey-Osterrieth Complex figure. For dementia specific tests suggested are: Clinical Dementia Rating and Dementia Rating Scale.

There is a plethora of memory tests in the market. It is important to select tests on the basis of referral from the neurologists/neurosurgeons. Level of intelligence and level of learning abilities contribute to the efficiency of memory. Intelligence is highly correlated with memory. WMS-1V is routinely administered to assess memory. At the same time simple sentences can be administered to measure memory at lower level. Memory tests are very many and each one has relevant value in testing the memory and learning abilities. Simple tests to assess concentration and memory are memory to recall numbers and recall simple words. Read out numbers like 754; one number per second. Do not hurry through the numbers challenging the patient. If an AD patient can repeat three numbers it is considered to be good. Other tests include phrases, sentences or lengthy passages.

One of my favorite tests is CVLT-California Verbal Learning Test. CVLT is meant to evaluate multiple cognitive abilities; ability to process verbal material and how they are retained within the frame of reference in terms of everyday memory task. A list consits of 16 items are presented to the patient to learn. CVLT comprises four categories. They come under clothing, spices/herbs, tools and fruits. CVLT is used to measure: immediate recall, short delay free recall; short delay cued recall; long delay free recall; long delay cued recall; long delay recognition. similar tests used are: rey auditory verbal learning test (RAVLT); and the verbal section of repeatable battery for the assessment of neuropsychological status (RBANS) (Wikipedia Encyclopedia). The test is standardized by Delis, D.C., Kramer, J.H., Kaplan, E., and Ober, B.A. (2000).

Other tests in use are the following:

- California Verbal Learning Test
- Cambridge Prospective Memory Test (CAMPROMPT)
- MCI Screen
- Memory Assessment Scales (MAS)
- Rivermead Behavioral Memory Test
- Test of Memory and Learning (TOMAL)
- Wechsler Memory Scale (WMS)
- Test of Memory Malingering (TOMM)

Cambridge Prospective Memory Test (CAMPROMPT) was stardardized by Barbara Wilson et al. (2005). The test assesses difficulties in prospective memory. It is an objective and standardized clinical instrument offering insights into a client's prospective memory or his/her ability to remember to do things at a particular time or within a given interval of time.

The Rivermead Behavioral Memory Test assesses everyday memory difficulties. Can the patient remember the news of the day? Is the patient oriented to time, place and person? Is the person capable of remembering daily activities?

The Memory Assessment Scales (MAS)

The MAS consists of 12 subtests based on the following seven memory tasks: verbal span, list learning, and memory for prose, visual span, visual recognition, visual reproduction and names-faces.

Test of Memory Malingering (TOMM)

This test is administered to discriminate between malingering and true memory impairments. Data is compiled on three different groups; those older people with cognitive abilities intact, cognitively impaired but not demented and with dementia. It is a 50-question visual memory recognition test that discriminates between true memory impairment and malingering (Wikipedia Encyclopedia). The test was standardized by Gordon Teichner and Mark T. Wagner (2004).

Automatism

Adults are able to repeat KG poem like "Jack and Jill Went Up the Hill" to fetch a pale of water with no effort. Adults are able to count automatically and even do multiplication effortlessly. ADIs in advanced stages will have difficulty with tests of this order.

Span/Supra Span Test

Patients are administered sequences to recall that exceed their working memory span, usually by about two items. The sequence involves a short-repeating sequence among the non-repeating items.

Brief Word-Learning Test

Three words are given to a patient with instructions that he/she will be asked to recall later. The mental status examination includes several aspects of memory and cognitive factors. The test then was extended to test memory. Two words are given together and later to remember the second word when the first word is mentioned. Example: Chennai—a city; rose—a flower; carrot—a vegetable; orange—a fruit.

One of the tests that is of repute with neuropsychologists is REY Auditory-Verbal Learning Test (AVLT) (Rey, 1964; E.M. Taylor, 1959). It evaluates short-term auditory-verbal memory, rate of learning, learning strategy, retroactive and proactive interference, memory process and so on.

Another variant to the AVLT is the Pictorial Verbal Learning Test (PVLT).

Sentence Recall

This test attempts to test attention span and short-term memory. Patients tend to remember what is presented to them initially—the primacy effect.

Story Recall

While patients may perform better on sentence recall, it is difficult for them to remember stories. Scoring the story is difficult because only few people can remember the story in full. The famous story is the Cowboy story. It is so humorous that patients remember most of the story. ADIs may leave most of the details. The gist of the story is: A cowboy in his cowboy outfit arrived in town with his dog. He went into a store leaving the dog outside. Cowboy changed his cowboy outfit. He bought a formal wear. The dog mourned and did not recognize him. So he changed into his cowboy dress. The dog was happy.

Benton Visual Retention Test (BVRT)

This test involves so many different capacities: visuospatial perception, visual and verbal conceptualization, immediate memory span. Benton developed the test to provide a shorter assessment for immediate non-verbal memory to supplement the popular digit span test, and selected a format that was resistant to both emotional and subject-tester influence. The test was published in 1946, and is now currently in its 5th edition (Wikipedia encyclopedia).

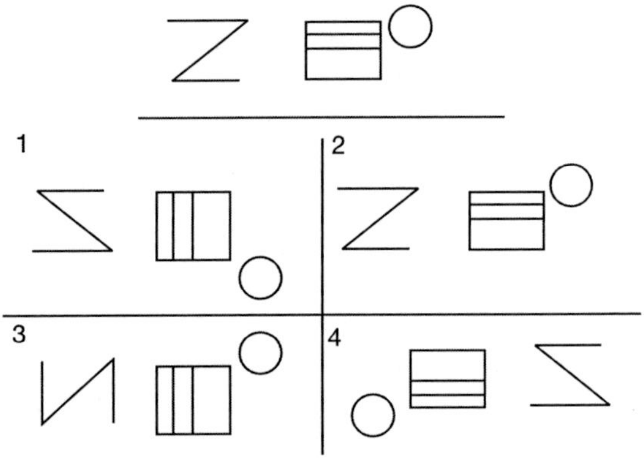

A sample design used in Administration M of the Benton Test. The original design is shown at the top, and after a delay, the four design choices are shown and the subject is asked to choose the one that best matches the original design.

The Benton Visual Retention Test is composed of three sets.

Ray-Osterrieth Complex Figure Test (ROCF) by Paul-Alexandre Osterieth 1994.

The test measures visuospatial abilities, memory, attention, planning, and working memory. The test has too many details and knowingly administering this test to an elderly may be done only after careful considerations. The test requires dynamic organization, memory for details and requires eyehand motor coordination and an understnding of geometry. It is a complicated line drawing. Many different cognitive abilities are needed for a correct performance, and the test therefore permits the evaluation of different functions such as visuospatial abilities, memory, attention, planning, and working memory and executive functions.

Drawings of geometric figures have been used to study the performance of patients with brain injury. One that is commonly used is the Bender Gestalt Test. Another is the Minnesota Percepto-Diagnostic Test.

Other variations are figure drawing, free drawing, copying figures from mirror imaging, line drawing. On line drawing the patient is asked to close the eyes and draw over it. The right hemisphere patients generally perform inadequately on the drawing tests. One test alone should not be used to predict brain impairment since each lobe has its specialty.

Building and Assembling

The building tests involve, organization, planning, conceptualization and motor execution. Construction engineers that I tested who were under different types of stress could complete the task but with slow reaction time. Benton has series of articles on this topic. Wechsler included two-dimensional block design but Benton later devised three-dimensional block design. Object assembly subtest of WAIS-R highly correlates with block design. Critchley (1953) studied the parietal lobe extensively and concluded the importance of right parietal lobe in constructional activities.

Concept Formation

Concept formation is a process by which a person learns to sort specific experiences into general rules or classes. With regards to action, a person picks up a particular stone or drives a specific car. With regard to thought, a person appears to deal with classes (*Encyclopedia Britannica*).

These tests on concept formation focus on the quality or process of thinking. The answers are not right or wrong but whether the answer is abstract or concrete. Proverbs and interpretation of proverbs are tested to evaluate the nature of thinking. The younger generation is not familiar with proverbs. However, proverbs are included in some of the intelligence tests. For example, "A barking dog does not bite". Patients may interpret the proverbs explaining the proverb in concrete terms and schizophrenics may give a new meaning to it altogether. Instead of similarities of words, comparisons of two words are also used as a test to evaluate brain impairment.

Other methods are the method of finding difference between verbal concepts. This is introduced by A.L. Christensen in 1979. He introduced variations to this method. For example, when flower is mentioned the subject has to respond with the name of a flower. He also introduced the method of stating opposites. For example, "heathy-sick" Reitan and associates studied concept formation and eventually introduced the category test. This test has 208 items; which is bit too long for many patients and tested their patience.

Raven's Progressive Matrices (RPM) (Raven 1960): "Raven's Colored Progressive Matrices (RCPM) test is used to measure visuo-perceptual skills as well. This is a matching task. The patient is required to choose items that will match centrally presented stimuli. The possible matches are displayed in different areas of the visual scanning for the correct match. It has been used for neuropsychological studies.

Sentence arrangement (Kaplan, Fein et al. 1991): The individual words of a Sentence are laid out in a scrambled order with instructions to rearrange them. "Driver to pick up is his mother going."

Picture arrangement is based on concept formation and Reasoning. (WAIS-R).

Picture Completion Sub-test included in WAIS-R: Picture completion test requires visual recognition, and abilities to visually organize. The patient has to find the right parts to complete the picture.

Pictures can be used to study how a person reacts to situations emotionally, socially, intellectually and ideationally. Rorschach Test Cards are presented to patients and instructed to report as to what they see in those pictures and where in the cards. In describing the responses, the patient is likely to use colors and details. The details given by brain impaired patients are limited and confabulation may take place. A few may respond with perplexity.

Arithmetic Reasoning Problems: Difficulties in solving math problems may indicate brain impairment. In some cultures like India most people are good at math. Early rigorous training in math may stand in good stead even under adverse circumstances. Accountants that I have tested completed the arithmetic subtest of WAIS-111 quite well even after brain insults. Wide Range Achievement Test (WRAT) is handy to test mathematical abilities. Calculations may go wrong in the presence of brain impairment.

Executive function is a set of mental processes that helps connect past experience with present action. People use it to perform activities such as planning, organizing, strategizing, paying attention to and remembering details, and managing time and space. There are several models of executive functions (refer to Wikipedia encyclopedia). Theories of the executive system were largely driven by observations of patients having suffered frontal lobe damage. They exhibited disorganized actions and strategies for everyday tasks (a group of behaviors now known as dysexecutive syndrome), although they seemed to perform normally when clinical or lab-based tests were used to assess more fundamental cognitive functions such as memory, learning, language, and reasoning. It was hypothesized that, to explain this unusual behavior, there must be a system that co-ordinates other cognitive resources (Wikipedia encyclopedia). Stroop Test and Wisconsin Card Sorting tests are used to assess executive functions.

Delis-Kaplan Executive Function System (from Wikipedia encyclopedia) consists of nine tests.

This measure consists of the following subtests:

1. The Trail Making Test measures flexibility of thinking on a visual-motor sequencing task.
2. The Verbal Fluency Test measures letter fluency, category fluency, and category switching.
3. The Design Fluency Test measures one's initiation of problem-solving behavior, fluency in generating visual patterns. Creativity in drawing new designs, simultaneous processing in drawing the designs while observing the rules and restrictions of the task, and inhibiting previously drawn responses.
4. The Color-Word Interference Test measures ability to inhibit a dominant and automatic verbal response.
5. The Sorting Test measures concept-formation skills, modality-specific problem-solving skills (verbal/non-verbal), and the ability to explain sorting concepts abstractly.
6. The Twenty Questions Test measures the ability to categorize, formulate abstract, yes/no questions, and incorporate the examiner's feedback to formulate more efficient yes/no questions.
7. The Word Context Test measures verbal modality, deductive reasoning, integration of multiple bits of information, hypothesis testing, and flexibility of thinking.
8. The Tower Test measures spatial planning, rule learning, inhibition of impulsive and perseverative responding, and the ability to establish and maintain instructional set.
9. The Proverb Test measures one's ability to form novel, verbal abstractions.

These nine subtests generate 16 main achievement scores and hundreds of optional error, contrast, accuracy, and time-interval scores. As such, use of the computerized scoring assistant makes scoring the measure less time consuming.

Perseveration: An aunt of mine continuously states "everything is going wrong", "No hope" especially in the evenings. This may be due to sundowning but in the morning she is able to participate in normal conversations but conversation is very limited. She is 95 years of age, yet her memory is good so also her intelligence. At times she states "I cannot remember many events in my life". Her reading is limited now because of her diminished eyesight. She used to be a book worm. The perseveration in this case may be due to depression and should not be confounded with Alzheimer's.

Numerous Neuropsychological Tests are available today to assess neuropsychological disorders. An astute neuropsychologist can select the tests to befit the patient and the referral issues.

Neuropsychological Tests and the subtests will provide models to practice with to improve cognitive abilities. Memory clinics use models of these tests. These types of tests will help the caregivers and the patients to get involved in solving the problems raised by these tests. The problems make people think and find strategies to solve them. These exercises keep the brain active lest boredom and inactivation further damage the brain cells. Planned and streamlined activities for each AD patient will keep him/her from further deterioration.

Space and spatial perception: Both spatial disorientation and visual scanning defects may be involved in impaired judgment of distances. AD patients will have difficulties in this area and can get lost if they are left to themselves. ADIs have difficulty estimating distance. Patient can be asked to estimate the distance between self and an object in the room. The neuropsychologist can find various methods to train a patient so that the disparity in distance estimation can be improved. Difficulties with distance estimation can endanger them in many ways. Accidents can happen within the home itself. Kitchen can be a dangerous place for them. In order to improve the ability in spatial perception, place two objects at certain distance and ask them to estimate the distance. In other examples, the patient has to indicate when two objects were equidistant from each other. Moderately impaired AD patients will have difficulties to estimate the distance between moving cars on high way. The distance estimation tasks can be demonstrated and tested in the office of the neuropsychologist. Spatial orientation is one of the components of visual perception. There is a test known as Pencil-paper test to assess right-left orientation (D. Alexander, 1976). Intelligence teaser tests are found in *Young World* published by Hindu Newspaper in Chennai. Mild ADIs are able to perform this test within acceptable range of Right-Left Orientation. Currently, Google gives road map and all the information one needs on cell phones. Despite that people with left-right orientation issues make mistakes and make wrong turns on the roads.

The Mini-Mental State (MMSE)

It has relevance if used with other tests. Some are in a hurry to diagnose brain impairment with this screening test. Sample questions are: 1. Orientation to time: What is the date? 2. Registration: I am going to say three words. You repeat after I stop. Here they are: lion, apple, desk. Examiner can use any three simple words but familiar to the patient. (Repeat up to five times, but score only the first trial.) 3. Naming: What is this (point to a familiar object-Pen). A total score of 27/30 is normal. This is a quick screening test. Validity issues are raised on this test. It is now replaced by Modified Mini Mental Exam (3Ms) Montreal Cognitive Assessment (MOCA): It is useful as a quick measure of Mild Cognitive Impairment (MCI). It is stated that it is a good test to use for screening, diagnosis and tracking of mild Cognitive impairment; not for advanced stages of Alzheimer's Disease.

Porteus Maze was popular with psychologists in the 1960s. It is a good test to find out how a person conceptualizes the test and how a person plans to reach the goal through the maze. The test is hardly used now. The newspapers like *Hindu* and *Times of India* add semblances of these tests for people to exercise their brain in the morning while reading the news.

Bender-Gestalt Test is provided to a patient to draw the diagrams. The end-product will suggest the difficulties a patient has in conceptualization and organization. Some may not be able to draw angles and may leave details. Some may create something new depending upon the case in question. This test is used to test visual memory as well. The psychiatric patients and normal children whom I have tested invariably converted the dots into small circles. (I guess it is easier to do that.)

There are several tests to assess different aspects of the brain and its functions. There are several scales to measure dementia, and some neuropsychologists use them and some do not. In addition to neuropsychological evaluation, it is only sensible to evaluate the psychological status of the patient using MMPI 2. This test is too long for AD suspected patients or even elderly, profile of mood states, and so on. Rorschach in the hands of highly trained neuropsychologists can be administered on brain impaired patients. Currently, elaborate evaluation by a neuropsychologist is not necessary because of the advanced technological devices used in the identification of brain disorder.

Some of the other test that is used by experimental psychologists to test concentration is: Vigilance Test. In experiments the subjects are asked to tap when a green light is shown and not to any other color lights. This is used by department of transportation in USA.

To repeat the digits is another way to test vigilance. This can be made gradually more difficult like the number 5, 2, 6 stand for E s u. Another efficient test is PASAT. It tests the skill of adding numbers and concentration.

The Digit Vigilance Test (**DVT**) is standardized by Ronald F. Lewis. The test is sold by PAR. It is a simple task designed to measure vigilance during rapid visual tracking and selection of target stimuli. Respondents are asked to find and cross out either sixes or nines, which appear randomly within 59 rows of single digits on two separate pages.

The Clock Drawing Test (CDT) is widely used in clinical neuropsychological practice. The CDT has been used traditionally to test "parietal lobe" but most empirical work on the CDT has focused on its sensitivity and specificity for detecting and differentiating subtypes of dementia, and there are surprisingly few studies of its neuroanatomical correlates.

Cancellation Tests: There are several cancellation tests. One is to cancel certain alphabets from a sheet that is presented with several alphabets and in some cases the alphabets may be mixed with numbers.

Stroop Test by J.Ridley Stroop (1935). In psychology, the Stroop effect is a demonstration of interference in the reaction time of a task. When the name of a color (e.g. "blue," "green," or "red") is printed in a color not denoted by the name (e.g. the word "red" printed in blue ink instead of red ink), naming the color of the word takes longer time and is more prone to errors than when the color of the ink matches the name of the color (green, red, blue, purple, blue, purple). All these are in their representative colors. The cognitive mechanism involved in this task is called directed attention. One has to manage attention, inhibit or stop one response in order to say or do something else. Stroop Test is used by neuropsychologists to identify brain impairment. The test has been modified throughout the years. The test combined with Word Fluency Test is a good test to diagnose left frontal lobe. A test akin to this is On Line. The test is based on speed of processing theory and selective attention Theory. There are three variations to this test. Luminosity, Cambridge brain science that is recently released and some of the on line tests use this model.

Visual Search and Attention Test (**VSAT**) by Max R. Trenerry, Bruce Crosson and others The VSAT consists of four visual cancellation tasks that require the respondent to cross out letters and symbols that are identical to a target. The test is sold by PAR. Parasuraman, R.; P.M. Greenwood et al. (2000) commented that the difficulties could be due to visuospatial difficulties of ADIs.

Other tests akin to the test are: Letter and Symbol Cancellation Test and Line Bisection Test.

The Span Tests: This comes in the format of number of digits, amount of information retained by a person to immediately report regarding what is seen and what is heard. Attention Span Test, 10 questions, five minutes.

Digit span: This is to repeat digits delivered for example 264 forward and backward. Normals score Digits forward 6 and backward 5. Interpretation of the difference between the two has to be interpreted with caution.

Earlier tests like Knox Cube Test: The examiner taps the cubes in a pre-arranged manner of increasing length and complexity and the subject must try to imitate the tapping pattern exactly. This test can be modified to train cognitive and motor abilities of AD. The WMS-R (Wechsler Memory Scale Revised) has a subscale known as visual memory span. It provides two cards on each of which eight squares are printed in a non-linear pattern, red for the forward span and green for backward span.Visual memory span measures attention span like the digit span which measures ability to concentrate to complete a task.

Sentence repetition: When ADIs are requested to repeat sentences be sure that the sentences are simple and short. In India there are 28 official languages. When sentences given are in English use very familiar words. For example, take this letter to your mother. Then the length of the sentence can be increased till the patient is not able to continue anymore.

Serial subtraction: This is part of Mental Status Exam. The patient is asked to subtract 7 from 100. I prefer to make it simpler for patients by asking them to subtract 3 from 50.

The Test of Sustained Attention and Tracking (TSAT)

Alphabet and counting backwards from 20. The test is made more complex by requesting the patient to count 1-A; 2-B and so on. The examiner has to keep in mind that the patient here is an ADI.

Paced Auditory Serial Addition Test (PASAT)

The patient has to add 60 pairs of randomized digits so that each is added to the digit immediately preceding it. On giving "2-8-6-1-9" and when called out 8 the Subject (S) calculates the numbers as 10, 14, 7, 10. The 8 is added to 2 + 10 and 8 + 6 is 14;

6 + 1 + 7 and 9 + 1 = 10. Each number is delivered at a speed of 1.2 seconds to 2.4 seconds. The PASAT was originally developed for use in evaluating patients with head injury (Wikipedia free encyclopedia). Later on O., Spreen and E., Strauss worked on this test. The test is stressful to a patient and hence better not to administer this test unless the examiner wants to test the limits. There are many ways to test attention without stressing out the patient. *Hindu* newspaper has variations of this test.

Trail Making Test (TMT)

Trails A and B Test is a neuropsychological test of visual attention and task switching. The test involves complex visual scanning with a motor component with motor speed and agility. This test has two parts Trail A and Trail B (show the design). Trail A consists of numbers. The individual has to draw lines to connect consecutively numbered circles on one sheet. On Trail B the individual has to connect numbers and letters alternatively for example start with digit 1 and then draw the line to connect A, and then 2 and connect to B, and so on. The test originally was used by US Army.

There are tests to measure visual inattention and visual neglect like the following:

Picture Description Tasks for Testing Visual Inattention

Pictures can be introduced to patients to describe the details of the pictures. Patients with lateralized lesions will neglect certain areas of the picture. I came across a workbook of 7-year-old. It is called junior writer. There is one picture depicting the kitchen and a woman standing in front of the kitchen sink. I showed this picture to an older person who has moderate memory disturbances.

To the question, 'In which part of the house is this person?' ,answer is 'Kitchen'. What is the lady in the picture doing? Answer: cooking. Where? "Cooking she answered whereas the lady is washing the vegetables at the sink. Is anyone helping her to cook? Not sure. She is perplexed. Then said this lady" (Same lady in the picture).

What are the vegetables that you can see in the picture? She is having problems to identify objects in the kitchen. Over all she has difficulty in naming the vegetables and has inattention to the right. She never identified the refrigerator that was on her right side. When a picture is presented to a patient to identify the parts and explain the parts some of them choose only one side of the picture to the exclusion of the other. This suggests a lateralized visual inattention to the opposite side.

Mr. A was working as a designer of crockery for a palace painted a large picture. He was a reputable artist. The left side of the picture was well detailed and meticulously done whereas he neglected the right side of the picture. The details were minimal and cohesion and order were faulty. He was in his 90s when he completed this picture. He had inattention to the spatial representation. Later he was diagnosed with a tumor in his right parietal lobe and AD.

Brain impaired people have difficulties to read maps and coin sorting. So these people will have difficulties in driving a car, shopping and marketing.

Color perception: Some individuals demonstrate difficulties to identify colors. Some people see almost every object in color. This is not an issue when you guide ADIs to do their activities.

Benton, neuropsychologist of University of IOWA Hospitals & Clinics has done extensive work with right hemisphere of the brain (Arthur Lester Benton, 1994) and contributions to Neuropsychological assessment by Arthur Benton et al. (1994).

Crichley published a book on parietal lobe in 1953. Crichley also pioneered the work on right hemisphere functions.

Test of facial recognition: This is a subtest included in most of the neuropsychological testing. Patients with right parietal deficits perform poorly.

Rorschach Technique

This is used as a personality assessment tool. In cases of brain impaired, the output is minimal and accuracy is inadequate to poor. Confusion and perplexity will be noted and lastly they will have slower reaction time. Perplexity is enormous on Card X. Some of them perceive many details with undefined percepts and some elaborate percepts. Some of the percepts do not carry any meaning.

Benton has reported the visuo-perceptive and visuo-constructive functioning in patients with brain diseases. Judgment of Line, three-dimensional construction are his outstanding contributions.

Auditory perception is tested with Speech Sound Perception Test. Some psychologists found that it is not a reliable test for left cerebral damage.

Seashore Rhythm Test: M. Sherer, O.A., Parsons, S.J. Nixon, R.L. Adams (1991): They felt that SSPT and SRT did not contribute much to neuropsychological battery. This is further supported by Boone, K.B., Rausch R.J. (1989).

Tactile Sensation: Sensations are routinely tested by neurologists. Neuropsychologists also conduct the test in their offices. A cotton ball is used on hands and face single and double simultaneous stimulation. Tests are conducted for touch, pain, pressure, temperature and muscle position sense.

There were other methods earlier in the history of experimental psychology. One was to determine which bottle with tiny lead balls is heavier than another comparatively. Trials are given informing the weight of each one of them. After trails, the bottles are placed in the palm of the S who is blind folded, to determine which bottle is heavier than the other. Most of the above tests have been tried first in the experimental labs.

Skin writing, fingertip writing are used to test tactile sensation. Touch sensation is very important in the case of an AD if she/he prepares food and in the kitchen. All precautions have to be taken to protect the person from harm.

Olfaction and taste are also tested since sensations diminish as people grow older.

THE WECHSLER ADULT INTELLIGENCE SCALE-1V SUBTESTS

Verbal Comprehension: Abilities Measured

Similarities: Measures abstract verbal reasoning. (In what way are dog and cat the same?)

Vocabulary: degree to which one has learned, been able to comprehend and verbally express and state meaning of words [*anecdote. On WISC when I asked a-14-year-old boy (USA), the meaning of the word Belfry he replied "The Bell rings and we all rush out and we are free" and he laughed. Even to-day I am amused about it.]

Information: Degree of general information acquired from culture. For example, who is the prime minister of United Kingdom, or India?

Comprehension: Ability to deal with abstract social conventions, rules and expressions.

Perceptual Reasoning. Subtests: Abilities Measured

Block Design: Spatial perception, visual abstract processing, and problem solving.

Matrix Reasoning: Non-verbal abstract problem solving, inductive reasoning, spatial reasoning.

Visual Puzzles: Spatial reasoning.

(*Picture Completion*): Ability to quickly perceive visual details.

(*Figure Weights*): Quantitative and analogical reasoning.

Working Memory, Core, Supposed Abilities Measured

Digit span: Attention, concentration, mental control.

Arithmetic: Concentration while manipulating mental mathematical problems.

(*Letter-number Sequencing*): Attention, concentration, mental control.

Processing Speed, Abilities Measured

Symbol search: Visual perception/analysis, scanning speed.

Coding: Visual-motor coordination, motor and mental speed, visual working memory.

(*Cancellation*): Visual-perceptual speed.

*The tests not in brackets are CORE subtests.

All these tests are timed.

Today the above-mentioned tests are used for academic purposes and not specifically for neuropsychological diagnosis. This test gives an IQ measure known as "Intelligence Quotient". Normal IQ is 100.

(Children's games these days are modeled after principles underlying these tests. Elderly people and Alzheimer's patients may want to practice with these types of games to keep cognitive abilities intact.)

There are four index scores representing major components of intelligence:

- Verbal Comprehension Index (VCI)
- Perceptual Reasoning Index (PRI)
- Working Memory Index (WMI)
- Processing Speed Index (PSI)

Two broad scores are also generated, which can be used to summarize general intellectual abilities.

Full Scale IQ (FSIQ) based on the total combined performance of the VCI, PRI, WMI, and PSI.

General Ability Index (GAI) based only on the six subtests that the VCI and PRI comprise.

WECHSLER MEMORY SCALE-1V (WMS-1V)

This new version of WMS contains the following subtests:

- Logical Memory I
- Logical memory II
- Verbal Paired Associates I
- Verbal Paired Associate II

- Design Memory I
- Design Memory II
- Visual Reproduction I
- Visual Reproduction II
- For older adults this test is modified. Administers only
- Logical Memory I and II
- Verbal Paired Associates I and II and
- Visual Reproduction Tests I and II.

Thus, indexes comprise only of Immediate Memory Index; Delayed MI; Auditory MI; Memory Index and Visual Memory Index. This is a flexible approach.

Areas of Assessment

There are changes made from WMS-Revised. Four subtests are added. They are:

- Spatial Addition
- Symbol Span
- Design Memory
- General Cognitive Screener

Three subtests retained with modifications:

Logical Memory: For people over 65-90 a new short story is introduced.

Verbal Paired Associates: This is modified to accommodate various age groups. For 65-90 years of age group there are 10 items. Out of which six items are hard. Scores for immediate versus delay and recognition versus delay can be obtained.

Visual reproduction with a few changes from WMS-revised is introduced in WMS-1V.

Several subtests were dropped from WMS-revised. New items are added. Eight subtests were discarded. They are: Information, spatial span, mental control, faces, digit span, family pictures, letter number and word list (*CVLT-II can be entered into Index).

For older people between the ages of 65 to 90 a short story is included. Story has only 14 items. These items are easy to remember and are familiar items.

Spatial Addition: Based on "N-Back Paradigm", spatial Addition requires minimal motor function. The client must remember location of dots on two separate pages.

1. Add or subtract locations
2. Hold and manipulate visual spatial information

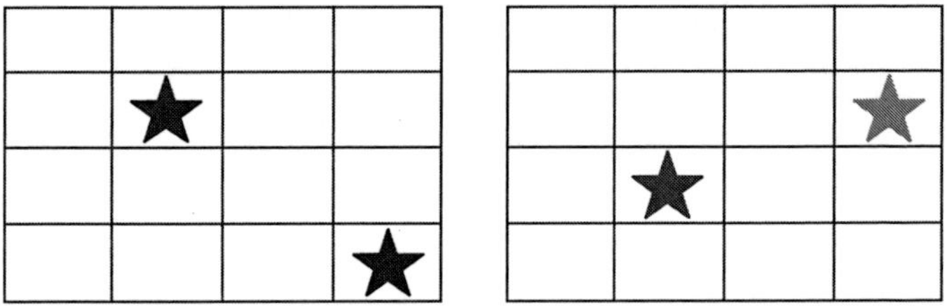

Symbol Span

"Visual Analog to Digit Span" clients are asked to remember the design and the left to right sequence of the design. The clients are then asked to select the correct design from foils and choose them in the correct sequence.

You can obtain scores for spatial, details, and correct content in the correct location as well as contrast scores for spatial versus detail, immediate versus delayed, and recognition versus delayed.

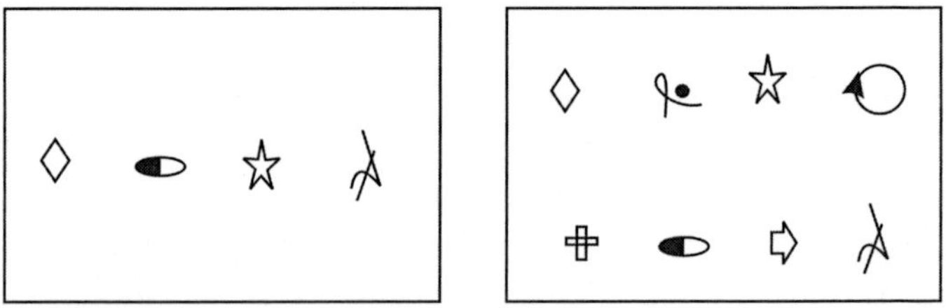

Design Memory

Containing four items of increasing difficulty, Design Memory evaluates:

Immediate and delayed recall as well as delayed recognition. It does not include drawing and reduces the opportunity to guess the correct response. The test obtains Scores for Spatial, details, and correct content in the correct location.

The Test has dropped a few of the subtests from earlier version. The authors paid special attention in the choice of tests for older people. Tests adopted are:

> LM I and II; Verbal Paired associate I and II and Visual Reproduction I and II: Symbol Span is added. Indexes are Immediate MI; Delayed MI; Auditory MI and Visual MI.

On Logical Memory for older adults Anna Thompson story is replaced with Ruth and Paul story. It has only 14 items whereas Anna has 25. The story is age appropriate and the language is very simple. The tests are age appropriate. The test findings can be used to detect MCI.

The new cognitive screener can be used to quickly evaluate significant cognitive impairment.

(*One of my friends at V.A. Hospital in Phoenix asked me why do you want to give all these tests when WAIS results can give you all the information you need? This test has been researched for several years and can be used to find the extent of brain impairment.) She may have a point.

AD affects every aspect of behavior. Cognitive changes are extensive in advanced cases. Concentration, learning and memory are deteriorated. They may not be aware of these changes taking place in their cognitive sphere. The ADIs gradually lose independence of reasoning and thinking. Consequences of deterioration in cognitive abilities restrict one from social interactions. Thus, this is a vicious circle. The more a person withdraws from human interactions, the less will be the verbal communication and usage of language functions. DeBettignies et al., 1990; Feher, Mahurin et al., 1991; McGlynn and Kaszniak, 1991; McGlynn and Schachter, 1989 have conducted research in this area. The Speech and Language department contributed the findings of their studies. Persons with dementia have trouble producing linguistic information since they have difficulties to think, and generate ideas. This is due to difficulties in information-processing and due to semantic memory disturbances.

Depression can play an important role in differential diagnosis. Some neuropsychologists have coined a term called Dementia Syndrome of Depression and Depression-related Cognitive Dysfunction (Stoudemire, Hill, Gulley and Morris: 1989). In my opinion, the pattern of memory disturbances between the two groups is different. On the other hand, if depression and dementia coexist, treatment of depression does not improve the features of dementia. Psychiatric symptoms will be present in dementia from anxiety, depression to schizophrenia. An astute neuropsychologist may be consulted to make the differential diagnosis.

In Alzheimer's, as in all cortical dementia memory difficulties are paramount. Kaszniak, Poon, and Reige; 1986 in the book *Neuropsychological Assessment of Dementia and Depression* discuss the nature of memory deficits.

Neuropsychological Tests and Neuropsychological Exam

Selection of Neuropsychological Tests

The battery of tests must cover: attention, concentration, learning, reasoning, verbal functions, and memory, visual perception, construction, concept formation, executive function, motor abilities and emotional status. Beyond this basic battery, other appropriate tests will be selected and administered to address the issues at hand. Neuropsychological tests must be selected to address all the relevant aspects of the case. The focus of clinical neuropsychology is the diagnostic assessment and intervention of individuals with organic or acquired neurocognitive deficits. The neuropsychologist must be relaxed during testing in order to make the patient at ease. Introduce the session with pleasantries but be professional, be supportive of the patients who are under psychological distress and with cognitive deficits. Interview must address all issues so that results and conceptualization of the results can be helpful to everyone involved with the case. Examine as to the onset of the symptoms and progress of the symptoms; educational and occupational history; tasks involved, details of the job; social history; family history and history of intellectual assessment if any, medical history, medications along with information with regard to significant past and current events and finally current living situations. In India people belong to different castes and one has to be sensitive to this issue. Be careful when enquiring into sensitive topics. Be very patient and encouraging of the patient while the testing is carried out. Do not show impatience. Observe the test behaviors very closely to get a better understanding of the patient. These observations will play a crucial role in the interpretation of the results and conceptualization of the patient.

The neuropsychological Report should incorporate the following: Reasons for the referral; Interview and Observations, the reasons for the selection of the Neuropsychological tests. The report should include presentation during assessment, results of tests explained with interpretations, conclusions and recommendations. The report should be succinct and keep in mind the main purpose of the assessment and how the results will be understood by the reader, not necessarily only by the neurologists and neuropsychologists; it could be read by physicians, nurses, occupational therapists, social workers, and other ancillary professionals. The patient may want to know the results. Be very careful how the information is imparted to the patient and close relatives. The clinical report must be complete and must depict a comprehensive picture of the neuropsychological deficits and strengths of the patient. The summary report must document all the cognitive domains tested; the personality tests administered if any, and additional information and additional findings, i.e. if additional psychological tests are administered. The report should conclude with summary and recommendations. In the summary, it is important to point out what the results indicate regarding the referral question. The recommendation's section should contain practical recommendations to assist the patient, family, treatment team and finally occupational/activity therapists and others involved with the management and treatment of the patient. Family of the ADIs may be involved in therapeutic endeavors.

Maintain high ethical standards. Confidentiality is very important. Get release of information duly signed. Consider functional issues and ADL functions. Consider tests for different functional areas if requested.

Categories of neuropsychological tests for neuropsychological Assessment.

- Intelligence
- Memory
- Language
- Executive function
- Visuo-Spatial and Visuo-Constructive
- Dementia specific
- Batteries assessing multiple neuropsychological functions.

For Intelligence

Wechsler Adult Intelligence Scale (refer to WAIS-IV for subtests and interpretations). There is a WAIS adapted for India.

Memory

Wechsler Memory Test IV for both verbal and visual.

For short-term memory for information and manipulation use any one of the following. This is left to the wisdom of the neuropsychologist.

- California Verbal Learning Test
- Cambridge Prospective Memory Test (CAMPROMPT)
- Memory Assessment Scales (MAS)
- Rey Auditory Verbal Learning Test
- Rivermead Behavioral Memory Test
- Test of Memory and Learning (TOMAL)
- Short sentences and stories.

Language

Language functions include speech, reading and writing, all of which can be selectively impaired. Some of the tests to assess are the following:

- Boston Diagnostic Aphasia Examination
- Boston Naming Test
- Comprehensive Aphasia Test (CAT)
- Multilingual Aphasia Examination.

Executive Functions

The executive functions include: problem solving, planning, organizational skills, selective attention, inhibitory control and some aspects of short-term memory. The following are the tests in the market:

- Behavioral Assessment of Dysexecutive Syndrome (BADS)
- CNS Vital Signs (Brief Core Battery)
- Continuous Performance Task (CPT)
- Controlled Oral Word Association Test (COWAT)
- Delis-Kaplan Executive Function System (D-KEFS)
- Digit Vigilance Test
- Figural Fluency Test
- Halstead Category Test; Ravens Progressive Matrices
- Kaplan Baycrest Neurocognitive Assessment (KBNA)
- Kaufman Short Neuropsychological Assessment
- Paced Auditory Serial Addition Test (PASAT)
- Rey-Osterrieth Complex Figure
- Ruff Figural Fluency Test
- Stroop Task
- Test of Variables of Attention (TOVA)
- Tower of London Test
- Trail-Making Test (TMT) or Trails A and B
- Wisconsin Card Sorting Test (WCST)

- Symbol Digit Modalities Test
- Test of Everyday Attention (TEA)
- Refer to the chapter on Neurological Testing for further selection of tests.
- Luria-Nebraska Neuropsychological Test.

Other tests that have been noted are:

ADAS-Cog (Alzheimer's Disease Assessment Scale-Cognitive) is better than MMSE.

Behavioral Pathology in Alzheimer's Disease Rating Scale (BEHAVE-AD).

CANTAB (Cambridge Neuropsychological Test Automated Battery): The test includes 13 interrelated tests of memory, attention and executive functioning like planning and sequencing to solve complex problems. The battery is administered through a computer. The test is sensitive to the early signs of Alzheimer's disease.

Neuropsychiatric Inventory (NPI): This test assesses 12 behavioral problems that commonly occur in people with AD and other dementias, including agitation, anxiety, apathy, delusions (fixed, false beliefs), hallucinations (sensing things that are not really there), euphoria (i.e. extreme happiness or elation), dysphoria (i.e. the opposite of euphoria), eating difficulties, loss of inhibition (the ability to hold back an extreme emotion or behavior), irritability, irregular motor behavior (e.g. shaking or trembling in just the hands or another body part and sleeping disturbances).

Neuroscientists continue to refine their understanding of the nature of executive control, and additional innovative procedures. Among a few first steps in that direction are non-veridical, actor-centered procedures such as the CBT (Cognitive Behavioral Therapy) and Iowa Gambling Test. Personality tests are available in short forms to elaborate ones like MMPI. Since the subjects under consideration are Alzheimer's patients, extensive clinical interview encompassing the information culled out from MMPI may be an option. In addition collateral interviews with immediate relatives and caretakers will give ample information regarding the mental status of the patient. Rorschach in the hands of experts can be a good tool to understand executive systems dysfunction in Alzheimer's patients. Well trained and experienced clinical/neuropsychologists will be able to get all the information needed on the basis of clinical interview and streamlined neuropsychological tests.

Ultimate question is how functional is this patient? and is this patient functional on Activities of Daily Living?

REFERENCES

Albert, M.L. (1973). A Simple Test of visual neglect. *Neurology*, 23, 658-64.

Arrigoni and De Renzi (1964). Constructional apraxia and hemispheric locus of lesions. *Cortex*, 1, 170-97.

Barbara, A., Wilson, Eve Greenfield, Linda Car, et al. (2008). Rivermead Behavioral Memory Test-Third Edition (RBMT-3) .

Barbara, A., Wilson, Agnes Shiel, Jennifer Foley, Hazel Emslie, Yvonne Groot, Kari Hawkins, Peter Watson: Cambridge Test of Prospective Memory (CAMPROMPT).

Bender-Gestalt Test (1938). By Lauretta Bender and Bender Gestalt second edition (2003). *Psych Corp*.

Benton, Arthur L. (1st September 1945). "A Visual Retention Test for Clinical Use". (BVRT) *Archives of Neurology and Psychiatry* 54 (3): 212.

Benton, Hamsher et al. (1983). Three Dimensional Construction Tests.

Bieliauskas, L.A. (1993a). *Journal of Clinical and Experimental Neuropsychology*, 15, 421-38. Cognitive and psychopathological change in degenerative disease in the elderly.

Blessed, Tomlinson, and Roth (1968). Blessed Dementia Scale BDS.

Boone, K.B., Rausch R. *Clin Psychol*. 1989 Jul. 45(4): 614-18. Seashore Rhythm Test does not discriminate between patients with right vs. left temporal lobe damage.

Critchley, M. (1953). *The Parietal Lobes*. London, UK.

Delis, D.C., Kramer, J.H., Kaplan, E., and Ober, B.A. (2000). California Verbal Learning Test. Second Edition. San Antonio, TX: Psychological Corporation.

Delis–Kaplan Executive Function System. *Psych Corporation* (2001) and From Wikipedia, the free encyclopedia, Nine tests.

DSM-IV: American Psychological Association, 750, First Street, NE., Washington, DC, 2002.

Gauthier, L., Dehaut, F., Joanette, Y. (1989). The Bells Test: A quantitative and qualitative test for visual neglect. *Int J Clin Neuropsychol*, 11, 49-54.

Gordon Teichner, Mark T. Wagne. *Archives of Clinical Neurology*, April (2004), pp. 455-64: The Test of Memory Malingering (TOMM).

Gronwall (1977). Cornwall and Sampson, (1974), p. 372: Paced Auditory Serial Addition Test Henrichs, R.W. (1990). Current and emergent applications of Neuropsychological assessment: Problem of Validity and Utility. *Professional Psychology: Research and Practice*, 21, 3, 171-76.

Halstead-Reitan Neuropsychological Test Battery (1977). The Category Test-Concept formation Tests in Visual Formats.

Kaplan, E. et al. (1991). Sentence arrangement.

Kaszniak, Poon, and Reige (1986). Memory deficits in the book *Neuropsychological Assessment of Dementia and Depression* edited by Martha Storandt and Gary R. VandenBos.

Kaszniak et al. (1987). Communication and Cognition in Normal Aging and Dementia.

Lamar, M., Zonderman, A.B., Resnick, S. (April 2002). *Neuropsychology*. 16(2):156-62.

Martha Storandt and Gary. *Neuropsychological Assessment of Dementia and Depression in Older Adults: A Clinician's Guide.*

Mattis, 1976, 1988. The Dementia Rating Scale (DRS).

Max R. Trenerry, Bruce Crosson, James DeBoe and William R. Leberisual. Search and attention test: Visual Search and Attention Test (VSAT) (published by PAR).

Memory Assessment Scale (1981-90). Test is sold by PAR.

M.M. (1985). *Principle of Behavioural Neurology*. Philadelphia: F.A. Davis.

MMPI (1930) by Starke R. Hathaway and J.C. McKinley, University of Minnesota and MMPI-2, revised in 2001, 2003, 2008 most recent one is known as MMPI-2 RF.

Money, (1976). Fig 9-4 Standardized Road-map Test of Direction Sense.

Parasuraman, R., P.M. Greenwood., G.E. Alexander (2000). "Alzheimer's disease constricts the dynamic range of spatial attention in visual search". *Neuropsychologia* 38 (8): 1126-35. Retrieved 19-11-2012.

Paul-Alexandre Osterrieth (1994). Ray-Osterrieth Complex Figure Test (ROCF).

Porteus, S.D. (1924). Porteus Maze.

Raven C. John (1936). Raven's Progressive Matrices. (Multiple choice intelligence tests of abstract reasoning.)

Rey (1964). E.M. Taylor. (1959). The Auditory-Verbal Learning Test (AVLT).

Ridley J Stroop (1935). Stroop Test.

Rouleau, I., Salmon, D.P., Butters, N. et al. Quantitative and Qualitative Analyses of Clock Drawings in Alzheimer's and Huntington's Disease. *Brain Cogn* 1992.

San Diego, Sattler (1992). Digit span and speed of memory psychology laboratory.

Sherer, M., O.A. Parsons, S.J. Nixon., R.L. Adams: *J. Clin Exp Neuropsychol* 1991 Sep Bigler (5): 741- Bigler Our data indicate that the SSPT (Speech-sounds Perception Test) and SRT (Seashore Rhythm Test) failed to discriminate left- and right-hemisphere.

Shulman, K.I., Gold, D.P., Cohen, C.A., Zucchero, C.A. (1993). Cloak Drawing and Dementia in the Community: A Longitudinal STUDY. *Int J Geriatr Psychiatry*. 8:487-96.

Tales, A., S.R. Butler, J. Fossey, I.D. Gilchrist, et al. (2002). "Visual Search in Alzheimer's Disease: A Deficiency in Processing Conjunctions of Features". *Neuropsychological* 40 (12):1849-57. Retrieved on 19-11-2012.

Troscianko (2002). "Visual Search in Alzhimers's Disease: A Deficiency in Processing Conjunctions of Features". *Neuropsychological* 40(12): 1849-57. Retrieved on 19-11-2012. Vermont, Memphis State and Hahnemann Universities.

Wechsler Adult Intelligence Test-111(1997) and 1V (2008) WMS-1V (2009): Published by Psych Corporation.

W.G. Rosen, Mohs and Davis (1984, 1986). Alzheimer's Disease Assessment Scale (ADAS).

Ziad Nasreddine in Montreal, Canada (1996). Montreal Cognitive Assessment (MOCA).

7

Current Treatment for Alzheimer's

So far there are no medications to cure Alzheimer's. Current medications can ameliorate and slow down the symptoms and improve the quality of life. The brain's communication system breaks down with the destruction of the neurons, synapses and thus the transfer of neurotransmitters. Finally, the brain cells die and consequently, the brain communication network becomes dysfunctional.

The following information is taken from G8 Conference on Alzheimer's and Alzheimer's Society (2013): The dementia guide: Treatments Fact sheet 401.

There are two types of medications: Cholinesterases and Memantine. Cholinesterase Inhibitors are prescribed to prevent the breakdown of acetylcholine and by keeping acetylcholine level high to promote learning and memory. Cholinesterase Inhibitors are the following: donepezil (aricept) galantamine (reminyl-Razadine); memantine (namenda or ebixa); rivastigmine (exelon); tacrine (cognex). The ones in brackets are the brand names. Tacrine is very rarely prescribed currently because of serious side effects. Donepezil, rivastigmine and galatamine prevent an enzyme known as acetylcholinesterase from breaking down acetylcholine in the brain. Increased acetylcholine improves communication between nerve cells. All three cholinesterase inhibitors work in a similar way. Physician will choose the best one for you.

Memantine (Ebixa or Namenda) blocks glutamate. Glutamate is released in excess when the brain cells are damaged. Memantine can protect brain cells by blocking the effects of excess glutamate.

Mixed results are obtained when cholinesterase were administered to control aggressive behaviors in Alzheimer's. Research is ongoing to test the efficacy of these medications and as to which one is most suitable to treat Alzheimer's.

The most frequent side-effects of donepezil, rivastigmine and galantamine are loss of appetite, nausea, vomiting and diarrhoea. Other side-effects include stomach cramps, headaches, dizziness, fatigue and insomnia. Side-effects can be less likely for people who start treatment by taking the lower prescribed dose for at least a month (see 'Taking the drugs' section).

The side-effects of memantine are less common and less severe than for the cholinesterase inhibitors. They include dizziness, headaches, tiredness, increased blood pressure and constipation.

It is important to discuss any side-effects with the doctor and/or the dispensing pharmacist.

None of these drugs are addictive. National Institute for Health Care Excellence (NICE) Guidelines explain everything that one has to know about medications, dosage and how to discuss symptoms with the treating physicians. NICE recommends the questions that the patient may ask the doctor. "The clinical care guideline on the care and treatment of people with dementia, which NICE publishes alongside its guidance, stresses that the severity of a person's dementia should not be determined by cognition scores alone (for example, Mini Mental State Examination), but by a more holistic view of the patient's condition."

The physicians explain the side-effects to patients. All the above medication have serious side-effects. New compounds under development target the amyloid pathway, tau phosphorylation, or acetylcholine levels, and it is hoped that they will not only improve symptoms but also slow disease progression or even lead to a cure.

Alzheimer's Society G8 Conference 2013: Factsheet 407

Above information was reviewed by: Dr. Rupert McShane, Department of Psychiatry, University of Oxford and Coordinating Editor, Cochrane Dementia and Cognitive Improvement Group, and Dr. Denise Taylor, Senior Teaching Fellow in Clinical Pharmacy, Department of Pharmacy and Pharmacology, University of Bath.

(**Note*: Download a PDF of Drug treatments for Alzheimer's disease http://www.alzheimers.org.uk/site/scripts/documents.php?categoryID=200264. Read more about the access to drugs campaign and find out how you can get involved. More about the access to drugs campaign and find out how you can get involved.)

Amyloid presence within mitochondria causes dysfunction in the early stages of Alzheimer's by attaching itself to a protein called amyloid binding alcohol dehydrogenase (ABAD). This produces toxins in the brain, ultimately damaging changes in the brain's memory capabilities. Scientists want to block this interaction by finding new medications. New doses and formulations of these medications mentioned above have recently gained FDA approval. New compounds under development target the amyloid pathway, tau phosphorylation, or acetylcholine levels, and it is hoped that they will not only improve symptoms but also slow disease progression or even lead to a cure.

General Information on Drug Treatments

The FDA (US) has approved two types of medications known as: Cholinesterases and Memantine. Cholinesterase Inhibitors are prescribed to: (i) Prevent the breakdown of acetylcholine, a chemical messenger important for learning and memory. This helps communication among nerve cells by keeping acetylcholine levels high. (ii) Delay worsening of symptoms for 6 to 12 months. Cholinesterase inhibitors are not a cure, but can treat some symptoms in some people. People with mild to moderate Alzheimer's may find that their condition improve by taking cholinesterase inhibitors. This could be a reason for the overall improvement in thinking, memory, communication or day-to-day cholinesterases activities. Others may find that their condition stays the same, when they would have expected to become less able with the progression of dementia. Some people may not notice any effect at all. This medication is well tolerated. If at all there is any side-effect, they include nausea, vomiting, loss of appetite and increased frequency of bowel movements.

Tacrine is very rarely prescribed currently because of serious side-effects. Some physicians prescribe Vitamin E to treat Alzheimer's since it is an antioxidant, a substance that may protect brain cells and other body tissues from certain chemical wear and tear. No one should take Vitamin E to treat Alzheimer's. Vitamin E at the high doses can increase the risk of death. It can also interact negatively with other medications. Vitamin E is not approved by FDA. There is no strong evidence that Folate, vitamin B6, and Vitamin B12 and Vitamin E prevent AD or slow the disease once it occurs. Further research is still needed to confirm how effective memantine is for treating behavioral and psychological symptoms and the evidence shows it is more effective than using antidepressants or anticonvulsants.

The other anti-dementia drugs—donepezil, rivastigmine and galantamine—are known as cholinesterase inhibitors. Cholinesterase inhibitors, particularly rivastigmine and donepezil, may reduce the severity of some behavioral and psychological symptoms in dementia and help delay their onset.

Amyloid's presence within mitochondria causes dysfunction in the early stages of Alzheimer's by attaching itself to a protein called amyloid binding alcohol dehydrogenase (ABAD). This produces toxins in the brain, ultimately damaging changes in the brain's memory capabilities. Scientists want to block this interaction by finding new medications. New doses and formulations of these medications mentioned above have recently gained FDA approval. New compounds under development target the amyloid pathway, tau phosphorylation, or acetylcholine levels, and it is hoped that they will not only improve symptoms but also slow disease progression or even lead to a cure" (Benek, O., Musilek, K., Kuca K PMID: 23251955 PubMed - indexed for MEDLINE.: Mitochondrial enzyme ABAD and its role in the development and treatment of Alzheimer's disease.)

Drug Treatments

All drugs have at least two names: a generic name, which identifies the substance and a proprietary (trade) name, which may vary depending upon the company that manufactured it. For example, Aricept is the trade name for the anti-Alzheimer's drug donepezil hydrochloride. Immediate results should not be expected in people taking drugs for behavioral and psychological symptoms as any benefits may take several weeks to appear. Drugs may also stop working. This is because dementia is a degenerative condition, so the chemistry and structure of the brain will change during the course of the illness.

These drugs work by regulating neurotransmitters, the chemicals that transmit messages between neurons. They may help maintain thinking, memory, and speaking skills, and may help with certain behavioral problems. However, these drugs don't change the underlying disease process, are effective for some but not all people, and may help only for a limited time.

Two Russian institutions, the Saint Petersburg Geriatric Medical-Social Centre and the Military Medical Academy, will take part in international clinical trials of a new drug known as Dimebon to combat Alzheimer's and other neurodegenerative brain disorders. The treatment has to start at the early stages. It is thought that the drug, administered intravenously, will break down Apolipoproteins, a fragment of which is called beta-amyloid and is stored in brain tissue causing gradual atrophy. Dimebon, also known as Latrepirdine, was approved as an antihistamine in Russia in 1983 but discontinued studies are conducted at Case Western Reserve University by Mark Smith and Racelle Doody. The latter stated that Dimebon treats the symptoms of the disease like other drugs. Cardiff University is currently conducting research on Dimebon. (There is disagreement amongst scientists over Dimebon.)

As to drug treatment it is important to be aware that all drugs have side-effects that may worsen symptoms. As side-effects are usually reelated to dosage, the doctor may start with a low dose which will be gradually increased until the desired effects are achieved. Once treatment has begun, it is important that it is regularly reviewed by the doctor. In the case of antipsychotic drugs, review should be carried out after six and/or twelve weeks. Drugs should always be taken exactly as prescribed by the doctor. Alzheimer's disease often affects the way people feel and act. The chief cause of behavioral symptoms is the progressive deterioration of brain cells. Medicines, environmental influences and some medical conditions also can cause symptoms or make them worse. Future Alzheimer's treatments may focus on combinations of medications like those used for many cancers and AIDS rather than a single compound. Future medications will attempt to target Beta-amyloid plaques. Two strategies aimed at Beta-amyloid include immunizing the body against it and blocking its production. Most current immunization studies focus on administering antibodies against Beta-amyloid from outside sources instead of enhancing a person's immune system. Another research effort is exploring the value of intravenous (IV) infusions of a product obtained from donated blood. This product contains naturally occurring antiamyloid antibodies from the donors. Researchers are investigating laboratory engineered monoclonal antibodies. Another treatment is the production blockers so that it reduces the amount of Beta-amyloid formed in the brain. Beta-amyloid is produced from a "parent protein" in two steps. This is performed by two different enzymes. Experimental drugs are administered to block the activity of the two enzymes. Another attempt is to keep tau from tangling and reducing inflammation in the brain. (Refer to current research as noted in the G8 conference on Alzheimer's.) Researchers are looking into why Alzheimer's causes chronic, low level brain cell inflammation and how to treat with non-steroidal anti-inflammatory drugs. Researchers are studying the effects of insulin on the brain and brain cell function and whether the insulin changes in the brain may be related to Alzheimer's. An insulin nasal spray is being tested to find out whether it slows or delays Alzheimer's progression. High blood pressure, heart disease, stroke, diabetes, high cholesterol are likely to be the causes for AD. The brain health is closely connected to heart health. Furthermore, a strong genetic Alzheimer's risk factor is one form of a gene from a protein that carries cholesterol in the blood (apolipoprotein E). What is good for the heart is good for the brain. This is being investigated. 1. Current drugs for heart disease risk factors: Researches are investigating whether drugs now used to treat high blood pressure, diabetes and high cholesterol may also help people with Alzheimer's or reduce the risk of developing the disease. 2. Drugs aimed at new targets: investigation into the connection between heart disease and Alzheimer's at molecular level and then find new drugs. Lifestyle changes are important. Developing new medications is a slow and painstaking process. To help accelerate this, the Coalition Against Major Diseases (CAMD), an alliance of pharmaceutical companies, nonprofit foundations and government advisers, have forged a first-of-its-kind partnership to share data from more than 4000 study participants. (The above information is from G8 Summit of 2013, Alzheimer's Society and Alzheimer's Association.)

Rudy Tanzi of Harvard Medical School has helped to create a drug called PBT2. It prevents the production of protein plaques and tangles that kill brain cells. "It also induces new neurons to grow in the hippocampus, which improves executive function," PBT2, a drug that's now in phase 2 clinical trials in Australia. Unlike the recently failed drugs, which use antibodies to attack Beta-amyloid, PBT2 takes a different approach. Certain metals in the brain (copper and zinc) help drive production of the plaques and tangles. PBT2 prevents this from happening. "It takes the metal away from the amyloid protein so it can't form plaques. It removes metal that was trapped and makes it available again for dozens of brain functions like gene activity and antioxidant health. PBT2 also keeps tangles from forming. And finally, "it induces new neurons to grow in the hippocampus, which should improve executive function," says Dr. Tanzi (Harvard Health Publications Harvard Medical School, Jan. 2013).

NeuroAD uses a non-invasive system of transcranial magnetic stimulation (TMS) and cognitive training to improve cognitive function in people with mild to moderate Alzheimer's disease. Patients solve computer exercises ranging from identifying colours, shapes, letters and animals to solving memory games. This technique improves cognitive abilities. Simultaneously, the very same regions of the patient's brain responsible for memory and learning receive electromagnetic stimulation which reactivates brain cell activity. Each Brain Stimulation is followed by a computer challenge. "It doesn't cure the disease, but it does make the brain circuits work better" states the lead researcher Dr. Alvaro Pascual-Leone, Professor of Neurology at Harvard Medical School. The only side effects so far have been mild headaches. And while the treatment is already approved in Israel and some countries in Europe, Dr. Pascual-Leone emphasizes the need for more studies.Trial participants undergo a MRI scan of the brain to pinpoint affected regions, and then receive five one-hour sessions per week for six weeks, in addition to long-term maintenance and follow-up. The treatment is painless and non-invasive, and can be repeated after its effects begin to wane. Consult a geriatric physician and a neuroscientist prior to brain stimulation.

Treatment of Alzheimer's 2014, 19 March; Facts and Figures by Alzheimer's Society: None of the pharmacologic treatments available today for Alzheimer's disease slows or stops the malfunction and death of neurons in the brain that cause Alzheimer's symptoms and eventually make the disease fatal. The available and recommended drugs temporarily improve symptoms of AD by increasing the amount of neurotransmitters in the brain. The effectiveness of this treatment varies from individuals to individuals.

As of now new treatments are in the horizon. Active management of Alzheimer's can improve the quality of life. The following are recommended by the Alzheimer's association. 1. Appropriate use of available treatment options; 2. Effective management of coexisting conditions; 3. Coordination of care among physicians, other health care professionals and lay caregivers; 4. Participation in activities and/or adult day-care programs and 5. Participation in support groups and supportive services.

2014 Facts and Figures recommend Non-Pharmacologic Therapy: Variety of non-pharmacologic therapies has been recommended and different nations have their own way of dealing with Alzheimer's. These modalities improve the quality of life and maintain cognitive reserve hopefully. Cognitive training, cognitive stimulation and training in activities of daily living appeared encouraging as an intervention.

Behavior change in ADIs is very discomforting to close relatives and family members. The behavior changes are due to progressive deterioration of the brain cells. Irritability, anxiety, depression, anger, aggression, general emotional distress, physical and verbal outbursts, restlessness, pacing and odd behaviors like staying on one topic at a particular time of the day may occur. Some may manifest psychotic features like delusions and hallucinations. Sleep disturbances is likely. Use of psychotropic medications is not specifically approved by FDA. However, physicians prescribe medications. One has to know the pros and cons of drugs. If one is placed on psychotropic medications, he should be monitored closely.

Medications

Antidepressants are prescribed for low mood and irritability; anxiety, restlessness, verbally disruptive behavior and resistance. Antipsychotic medications are prescribed for hallucinations, delusions, aggression, agitation, hostility and uncooperativeness.

Based on scientific evidence, as well as governmental warnings and guidance from care oversight bodies, individuals with dementia should use antipsychotic medications only under one of the following conditions:

- Behavioral symptoms are due to mania or psychosis
- The symptoms present a danger to the person or others
- The person is experiencing inconsolable or persistent distress, a significant decline in function or substantial difficulty receiving needed care.

Antipsychotic medications should not be used to sedate or restrain persons with dementia. The minimum dosage should be used for the minimum amount of time possible. Adverse side effects require careful monitoring.

Whom can Antipsychotic Drugs Help?

Drug trials have shown that, for people with Alzheimer's disease, antipsychotic drugs can have a small but significant beneficial effect on aggression and to a lesser extent, psychosis (delusions and hallucinations). These effects are seen when antipsychotic drugs are taken for a period of 6-12 weeks. The benefits of these drugs for other symptoms are limited and so also when used for longer than 12 weeks.

For mild-to-moderate behavioral and psychological symptoms, National Institute for Health and Clinical Excellence (NICE) England recommends that antipsychotic drugs should not be prescribed in the first instance. Non-drug treatments should be used before antipsychotics are considered. People with severe behavioral and psychological symptoms may be offered antipsychotic drugs in the first instance, but only in certain, clearly defined circumstances. Symptoms are considered severe if they are happening very frequently and causing a great deal of distress and risk to the person and others around them.

Issues associated with the Use of Antipsychotic Drugs in People with Dementia: Antipsychotic drugs help around half of the people with dementia that take them and can be an important part of their treatment. However, they can cause serious side-effects, especially when used for longer than 12 weeks. This is why all prescriptions should be monitored and stopped after 12 weeks, except in extreme circumstances. Drugs can be safely stopped after this period with no worsening of behavioral symptoms in most people. People should always consult their doctors first before they stop taking any medication.

Possible side-effects include:

- sedation (drowsiness)
- parkinsonism (shaking and unsteadiness)

- increased risk of infections
- increased risk of falls
- increased risk of blood clots
- increased risk of stroke
- worsening of other dementia symptoms
- increased risk of death.

It is important to consider that antipsychotic drugs may help reduce behavioral and psychological symptoms, but because of these side-effects, this may be at the expense of the person's quality of life.

There is evidence that people with dementia are inappropriately treated with antipsychotic drugs. For example, antipsychotic drugs are prescribed for an extended period of time and are prescribed to treat mild behavioral and psychological symptoms. It is thought that around two-thirds of antipsychotic prescriptions are inappropriate. Alzheimer's Society would like to see these drugs are used only when they are really needed.

Antidepressants and Anticonvulsants

Research suggests that drugs developed to treat depression (antidepressants) can also be an effective treatment for behavioral and psychological symptoms in dementia. Specifically, studies have shown that the antidepressant drugs sertraline and citalopram may help reduce agitation. Antidepressants may treat apathy which is thought to be the most common behavioral change seen in people with Alzheimer's disease. In addition to this, some psychotic symptoms may respond to the use of antidepressants. There is currently a need for more evidence about the effectiveness and safety of antidepressants and anticonvulsants in the treatment of behavioral and psychological symptoms in dementia. These drugs should not usually be combined with each other or with antipsychotics. Anticonvulsant drugs are used at times for symptoms of aggression and agitation (Alzheimer's Society, Depression and Anxiety).

Sleep Disturbances

Sleep disturbances are common among ADs. Many people with Alzheimer's experience changes in their sleep patterns. Scientists do not completely understand why this happens. As with changes in memory and behavior, sleep changes occur with the progression of Alzheimer's. Many older adults without dementia also notice changes in their sleep, but these sleep disturbances occur more frequently and tend to be more severe in Alzheimer's. There is evidence that sleep changes are more common in later stages of the disease, but some studies have also found them in early stages. Sleep changes in Alzheimer's may include difficulty to stay asleep and thus may get out of bed and wander or pace.

Drugs Used to Treat Sleep Disturbance

People with dementia often experience sleep disturbances including not being able to get to sleep and waking up throughout the night. Sleep disturbances may be made worse by many of the drugs commonly prescribed for people with dementia. Drugs can cause nightmares and excessive daytime sedation, meaning that the person is less tired at night. Increased stimulation during the day, avoiding daytime napping and avoiding caffeinated drinks late at night will help reduce sleep problems. If the patient takes dementia medication at night and is having problems sleeping due to nightmares or vivid dreams, then the alternative is to take the medication in the morning. Exercise and some complementary therapies such as bright light therapy, might also be helpful. If sleeping tablets (hypnotics) are prescribed, it is likely that these will be one of the newer tablets such as zopiclone or zolpidem, which generally don't make people feel unwell. It is also possible that people will be prescribed a sedative antidepressant instead of sleeping tablets such as trazodone. If the patients and their physicians feel that medication would be a good option, the tablets taken should meet their specific needs. For example, some hypnotics last only for a short duration. These tablets are most useful for people who have trouble falling asleep. Longer lasting tablets are more useful for people who find it hard to stay asleep.

Issues to Consider when Treating Sleep Disturbance

- If excessive sedation is given at bedtime, the person may be unable to wake up to go to the toilet and incontinence may occur—sometimes for the first time.
- If the person does wake up during the night despite sedation, increased confusion and unsteadiness may occur.
- Hypnotics should only be used on a short-term basis (less than two weeks), and so are best used intermittently, for example, when the care giver and person with dementia feel that a good night's sleep is necessary for either or both of them.
- The use of hypnotics should be monitored by the doctor.
- It is important to have realistic expectations about what duration of sleep should be expected. Older people rarely sleep for more than five to six hours at night, and in people with dementia this will often be spread out over a full 24 hours.

Daytime Napping and Other Changes in the Sleep-wake Cycle: Individuals may feel very drowsy during the day and then be unable to sleep at night. They may become restless or agitated in the late afternoon or early evening, an experience often called "sundowning". Experts estimate that in later stages of Alzheimer's, individuals spend about 40 per cent of their time in bed at night awake and a significant part of their daytime sleeping. In extreme cases, people may have a complete reversal of the usual daytime wakefulness-nighttime sleep pattern. Medical factors can contribute to sleeplessness. Restless legs syndrome, a disorder in which unpleasant "crawling" or "tingling" sensations in the legs cause an overwhelming urge to move them, thereby disturbing sleep. Sleep apnea, an abnormal breathing pattern in which people briefly stop breathing many times a night can result in poor sleep quality.

Non-drug Treatments for Sleep Changes

Non-drug coping strategies should always be tried before medications, since some sleep medications can cause serious side-effects. To create a healthy sleeping environment, the following may be considered:

- Maintain regular times for meals and for going to bed and getting up
- Seek morning sunlight exposure
- Encourage regular daily exercise, but no later than four hours before bedtime
- Avoid alcohol, caffeine and nicotine
- Treat any pain.

If the person is taking a cholinesterase inhibitor (tacrine, donepezil, rivastigmine or galantamine) avoid giving the medicine before bed.

- Make sure the bedroom temperature is comfortable; the bed and bed sheets are comfortable and pleasing to the patient
- Provide night lights and security objects
- Discourage staying in bed while awake; use the bed only for sleep
- Discourage watching television during periods of wakefulness.

In many cases, the patient's behavior is a reaction to an uncomfortable or stressful environment including inability to communicate, unfamiliar surroundings and overall unfamiliarity. Loud noises, frantic environment and physical discomforts are reasons for disorientation. Environment must be soothing and calm. Modify environment to reduce potential stressors that can create agitation and disorientation. Treatment staff has to keep calm themselves. Keep a regular sleep schedule. Increased physical activity during daytime will help a good night sleep. Bright light and taking Melatonin lessen the progression of dementia, improve sleep and overall improve general behavior.

Some people may prefer soft music that lulls them to sleep. Parallel to Western classical music, in south India people enjoy Carnatic music and songs from movies. Interaction with others must be encouraged but do not pressurize the reluctant patient.

Mostly people in India socialize with their own extended family and close friends. They often visit the patients. Children from the same family can be very therapeutic to patients.

Wandering may be due to restlessness and disorientation. Restlessness could be due to physiological needs like hunger or due to some specific need. Disoriented person needs reassurances. At times disorientation may be secondary to medications. Hallucinations and suspicion may be manifested by some ADs. Hallucinations can be the result of failing senses. Keep the environment calm and pleasant. Violent movies or television can contribute to paranoia. So do not allow ADs to watch emotionally disturbing movies. Do not get into a debate with a patient about suspicions. ADs may be distracted with another activity.

Exercise is good to relieve tension. Regular walking, seated and standing exercises, holding on to a chair or any other that is comfortable for the patient. This exercise is called chair aerobics. Re-engage the patient to some of the past hobbies and encourage the patient to take part in daily activities when possible.

Alzheimer's treatments currently work by temporarily improving symptoms of memory loss and problems with thinking and reasoning. These treatments boost performance of chemicals in the brain that carry information from one brain cell to another. However, these treatments don't stop the underlying decline and death of brain cells. As more cells die, Alzheimer's continues to progress.

Experts are cautiously hopeful about developing Alzheimer's treatments that can stop or significantly delay the progression of Alzheimer's. A growing understanding of how the disease disrupts the brain has led to potential Alzheimer's treatments that short-circuit fundamental disease processes.

> Drugs used to relieve behavioural and psychological symptoms in dementia (download a PDF of drugs used to relieve behavioural and psychological symptoms in dementia) (Alzheimer's Society).

Further Reading

Alzheimer's Society has published a booklet, reducing the use of antipsychotic drugs: A guide to the treatment and care of behavioural and psychological symptoms of dementia (code 864). Download from alzheimers.org.uk/antipsychotics or order a copy from Xcalibre on 01628 529240.

For details of Alzheimer's Society services in your area, visit alzheimers.org.uk/localinfo

The G8 Conference (2013): The Dementia Guide to Treatments.

Future Alzheimer's treatments may focus on combinations of medications like those used for many cancers and AIDS rather than a single compound. Meantime, the only NMDA receptor antagonist can be used as monotherapy as well as an adjuvant to ChEIs. New doses and formulations of these medications have recently gained FDA approval. New compounds under development target the amyloid pathway, tau phosphorylation, or acetylcholine levels, and it is hoped that they will not only improve symptoms but also slow disease progression or even lead to a cure.

(Dr. Tiedeman is ambulatory care clinical pharmacy specialist, Veteran Affairs Maryland Health Care System. Dr. Kim is geriatric clinical pharmacy specialist, Veteran Affairs Maryland Health Care System, Baltimore et al.)

Some of the new Alzheimer's treatments in development target microscopic clumps of the protein Beta-amyloid (plaques). Plaques have long been considered a sign of Alzheimer's disease.

Most current immunization studies focus on administering antibodies against Beta-amyloid from outside sources instead of enhancing a person's immune system. One large research effort is exploring the value of intravenous (IV) infusions of a product derived from donated blood. This product contains naturally occurring anti-amyloid antibodies from the donors. Other studies are investigating laboratory-engineered (monoclonal) antibodies.

Production blockers may reduce the amount of Beta-amyloid formed in the brain. Research has shown that Beta-amyloid is produced from a "parent protein" in two steps performed by two different enzymes. Several experimental drugs aim to block the activity of the two enzymes.

A vital brain cell transport system collapses when a protein called tau twists into microscopic fibers called tangles, which are another common brain abnormality of Alzheimer's. Researchers are looking at a way to prevent tau from forming tangles.

Reducing Inflammation

Alzheimer's causes chronic, low-level brain cell inflammation. Researchers are studying ways to treat inflammatory processes at work in Alzheimer's disease.

Studies in non-steroidal anti-inflammatory drugs have had varying results, but haven't confirmed treatment options and future developments.

> Geriatric psychiatrists should be consulted before any medication is prescribed. They may prescribe Tricyclic antidepressants, Benzodiazepines, sleeping pills, and antipsychotic medicines or may not prescribe any at all. Treatment goals are likely to change with Alzheimer's disease. Make sure you understand all the available options and the benefits and risks of each choice as your treatment plan evolves.
>
> Reviewed by: Dr. Rupert McShane, Department of Psychiatry, University of Oxford and Coordinating Editor, Cochrane Dementia and Cognitive Improvement Group, and Dr. Denise Taylor, Senior Teaching Fellow in Clinical Pharmacy, Department of Pharmacy and Pharmacology, University of Bath.

Most experts believe that additional genes may influence the development of late-onset Alzheimer's. Scientists around the world are searching for these genes, and have identified a number of common genes in addition to APOE E4 that may increase a person's risk for late-onset Alzheimer's. For more about this area of research, see the *Alzheimer's Disease Genetics Fact Sheet*.

A new study (*Huffington Post*, 03/19/2014) by Harvard scientists points to a possible answer, one that could spark further research that—ultimately—could lead to new drugs and treatments for dementia. Researchers have found that a protein active during fetal brain development, called REST, switches back on later in life to protect aging neurons from various stresses, including the toxic effects of abnormal proteins. But in those with Alzheimer's and mild cognitive impairment, the protein—RE1-Silencing Transcription factor—is absent from key brain regions. In laboratory tests, REST protected brain cells from dying when exposed to a number of stresses, including the Beta-amyloid protein that accumulates in the brains of Alzheimer's patients. Bruce Yanker said, One very positive, optimistic note from this study is that it suggests that dementia can be resisted by some people; it provides the first molecular inklings of how that might occur. The finding highlights a different approach to understanding neurodegenerative diseases instead of focusing on the negative changes that cause disease, researchers looked for lapses in the brain's protective mechanisms" (*Huffington Post*, 3/19/2014).

According to the research team led by Chen Gong at Penn State University, an abnormally high concentration of one inhibitory neurotransmitter was discovered in the brains of deceased Alzheimer's patients. Chen's team found that the GABA neurotransmitter was drastically increased in the deformed versions of the normally large, star-shaped "astrocyte" cells which, in a healthy individual, surround and support individual neurons in the brain. He said the research shows that the excessively high concentration of the GABA neurotransmitter in these reactive astrocytes is a novel biomarker that we hope can be targeted in further research as a tool for the diagnosis and treatment of Alzheimer's disease. A neurotransmitter present in deformed cells called "reactive astrocytes" that are located in the entry to the hippocampus, which is integral for memory and learning. GABA inhibition discovered in the study cannot be corrected by targeting amyloid proteins alone. The studies suggest that reducing the excessive GABA inhibition to the neurons in the brain's dentate gyrus may lead to a novel therapy for Alzheimer's disease. "Rescue of Alzheimer's Memory Deficit Achieved by Reducing Excessive Inhibition" (13 June, 2014). An ultimate successful therapy may be a cocktail of compounds acting on several drug targets simultaneously. The study was published in *Nature Communications* (June 14, 2014).

An article was published by the University of Southampton on June 18, 2014 under the heading "Self-Repairing Mechanism of the Adult Brain can Help to Preserve Brain Function in Neurodegenerative Diseases". The scientists at Southampton University have found that neurogenesis, the self-repairing mechanism of adult brain, can help to preserve brain function in neurodegenerative disease such as Alzheimer's, Prion or Parkinson's. The progress of Alzheimer's is viewed as unstoppable and irrevocable so far. But scientists at Southampton University reported that the brain has some self-repairing potential that accounts for the renewal of certain neuronal populations living in the dentate gyrus, a simple cortical region that is part of the larger functional brain system controlling learning and memory, the Hippocampus. This process is known as neurogenesis. The scientists have detected increased neurogenesis in the dentate gyrus that partially counteracts neuronal loss. While this self-repairing mechanism is effective in maintaining some neuronal functions at early and mid-stages of the disease, it fails at more advanced phases. The study is published in the journal *Brain*. (Diego Gomez-Nicola, Stefano Suzzi et al., "Temporal Dynamics of Hippocampal Neurogenesis in Chronic Neurodegeneration", *Brain*, June 2014).

A new drug called 2-PMAP reduced amyloid beta levels by 50 per cent. The research is conducted on rats. The news is released by NYU Medical Center as of June 3, 2014.

Environmental/Lifestyle Factors

Research also suggests that a host of factors beyond basic genetics may play a role in the development and course of Alzheimer's disease. There is a great deal of interest, for example, in associations between cognitive decline and vascular and metabolic conditions such as heart disease, stroke, high blood pressure, diabetes, and obesity. Understanding these relationships and testing them in clinical trials will help us understand whether reducing risk factors for these conditions may help with Alzheimer's as well. Further, a nutritious diet, physical activity, social engagement, and mentally stimulating pursuits can all help people stay healthy as they age. New research suggests the possibility that these and other factors also might help to reduce the risk of cognitive decline and Alzheimer's disease. Clinical trials of specific interventions are underway to test some of these possibilities.

Latest research. Up dates posted Jan. 8, 2014:

1. Stem cell model of familial Alzheimer's identifies New AD genes. Out of 14 genes, one gene is found to be the cause for inflammation.
2. Living brain cells created from Alzheimer's brain tissue.
3. Circadian Clock Proteins a Potential Therapeutic Target for Alzheimer's (Dec. 19, 2013).
4. New Tanzi Paper Identifies Two Late-Onset Gene Mutations (Sept. 20, 2013) and many more studies.

Neuroscientists of various universities of USA, England, Australia and some other countries are actively conducting research to find treatment for Alzheimer's.

Projects in England and USA are very many to record here. The following are some of them.

Novel drugs for treating Alzheimer's disease (University of St Andrews).

Testing the effect of the diabetes drug Liraglutide in Alzheimer's disease (Imperial College London).

How can we change stem cells into brain cells? (University of Nottingham).

Stimulating brain stem cells to repair damaged nerve cells (Institute of Psychiatry, Kings College London).

NIH 2011-2012 Alzheimer's Disease Progress-Report: Intensifying the Research Effort

Some of them are:

Understanding the Biology of Alzheimer's and aging brain.

Identifying genetic influences on risk for late-onset Alzheimer's, the most common form:

1. Detecting the earliest Alzheimer's-related brain changes, including further development of biomarkers to track the onset and progression of Alzheimer's.
2. Understanding gender and racial differences in the impact of Alzheimer's.
3. Stepping up translational research that enables the design and testing of new drugs.
4. Testing in clinical trials potential new therapies to prevent, delay, or treat Alzheimer's.
5. Finding better ways to support caregivers.

Alternative and Complementary Treatments of Alzheimer's with Herbs

When describing health approaches with non-mainstream medicines, people often use the words "alternative" and "complementary" interchangeably, but the two terms refer to different concepts:

Alternative therapy is a term usually used when a treatment is used in place of conventional medical care. An example of an alternative therapy is eliminating medications and using acupuncture and herbal supplements to treat Alzheimer's disease.

Complementary typically means that the approach or treatment is used in combination with traditional medical care. For example, an individual may be receiving both Exelon (Rivastigmine) and coconut oil.

The area of complementary and alternative medicine is controversial and changes regularly. Therapies that are considered 'complementary' or 'alternative' in one country may be considered conventional in another. Therapies that are currently considered alternative may become more mainstream over time, as researchers discover their effectiveness and they become integrated into mainstream health care practice. Some complementary and alternative therapies are now available in Western countries and other developed countries. There is little high-quality research into the treatment of dementia with complementary and alternative therapy. However, research on a number of therapies has provided some interesting preliminary results.

Ayurveda: According to Ayurveda, any disease related to the body and mind is the result of imbalance in Vata dosha. Moreover, Vata is responsible to maintain the balance among all the three doshas.

Tridosha is composed of Vata, Pitta and Kapha.

A dosha (dosa) is one of three bodily humors that make up one's constitution. These teachings are also known as the Tridosha theory. Well-balanced Vata dosha is necessary to maintain perfect health of the body and the mind.

Vata is the driving force behind balancing the Tridoshas. Imbalance of Vata triggers imbalance of both Pitta and Kapha.

Kerala Ayurveda Treatment (Kerala)[1]

Vata imbalances are common in old age. Ayurveda treats Alzheimer's by restoring Vata balance. Ayurvedic therapy for Alzheimer's starts with Vata balanced diet. Ashwagandha (*Withania somnifera*) powder with milk, ghee or skimmed milk is recommended to energize Vata.

Treatment of Alzheimer's Disease with Ayurvedic Medicine

Brahmi, Sankha Pushpi, Vacha, and Jatamansi are the main herbs used to treat brain disorders. Ashwagandharistha, Saraswatarishta, Smriti Sagaram, Maanasa Mitravati, Brahmivati, Kalyanaka Ghruta and other prepared medicine are available for AD treatment. The dosage for any one of these medicines is 20-50 gms per day.

Kerala Ayurveda recommends Pancha karma massages like Nasya Karma, Sirovasthi, and Dhara chikitsa for patients with brain disorders. It is stated that early diagnosis and proper medications with massages have better chances for cure.

(Kerala Ayurveda Limited[2] is a major force in health care, growing at a spectacular rate; new Ayurvedic Medicines).

Synchronized massage: It is beneficial to cure sleep disorders, and paralysis. Daily oil massage before bath is another important part of Alzheimer's treatment in Ayurveda.

Pizhichil treatment in Ayurveda is a combination of oil massage and heat treatment. This therapy was mostly used by Maharajas in the olden days, and popularly known as treatment for aristocrats. Cloth dipped in lukewarm medicated oil is squeezed over the patient's body uniformly and then the oil rubbed smoothly over the body of the patient by masseurs on either side. The session may take one hour including continuous oil applied over the body, massaging and stimulating the skin using hands and special cotton clothes. It is highly recommended for sleep disorders, rheumatic diseases, arthritis, paralysis, neurological disorders, blood pressure, nervous weakness and longevity.

Njavarakizhi can be considered as a contribution of Kerala to the field of Ayurveda. It is a method of treatment based on fomentation in which four boluses of a type of paddy (called Njavara, hence the name Njavarakizhi) with medicinal herbs are cooked in milk and the herbal decoction is made from Sida rhombifolia (Kurumthotti in Malayalam). Usually, there are two masseurs who start fomentation in an identical manner one from each side. The movement of hands has to be always from upwards to downwards and the Kizhi has to be kept always at a constant temperature. There are mainly seven positions in which the patient has to be during the fomentation process. Once the procedure has been completed, the medicinal paste is wiped off with palm leaf scrapers, followed by an oil bath. Njavarakizhi is used in the treatment of rheumatism, arthritis and other neuro-muscular disorders and for general rejuvenation of the body.

Ayurveda treatment approaches the patient as a whole by treating each of its parts in coordination. Treatment will often include any number of a variety of herbal concoctions, relaxation and meditative therapy, and changing of dietary and exercise habits. Through the integration of the proper changes in all aspects of life ayurvedic treatments restore balance to the whole individual. Daily oil massage before bath is another important part of Alzheimer's treatment in Ayurveda. Nutritious Ayurvedic foods like specialized rice preparations and Nervine tonics are beneficial for persons who experience the onset of or advanced stage of Alzheimer's disease. Ayurvedic cleansing processes (detoxification) like Panchakarma are not indicated for older people. Other mild cleansing techniques are used to purify body tissues.

Anil Kumar Singhal et al.[3] report that the following Medicinal plants have potentials to treat Alzheimer's. Some ayurvedic herbs like Guduchi, Liquorice, Padma, Vacha, Shankhpushpi, Goggulu, Amalaki (gooseberry), Musta Arjun, Ashwagandha, Galo Satva, and others are excellent herbs for slowing down the brain cell degeneration caused by Alzheimer's. They enhance the brain's ability to function, and therefore, provide stability when used consistently. These herbs are good to improve memory and aid in efficient learning.

Turmeric, Bacopa, Ginkgo Biloba are known herbs for Alzheimer's treatment. Ginkgo Biloba is known for its ability to enhance blood circulation. Its action is directly related to the vascular relaxing activity. Thus, Ginkgo can lower blood pressure and inhibit platelet aggregation. Scientific studies have shown its promise on Cognition-enhancement, if used during the early stages of Alzheimer's disease.

Other herbs recommended for cognitive enhancement in Alzheimer's patients are as follows: *Salvia officialis*, Rosemary, German Chamomile, lemon balm. Huperzine-A significantly improves memory, concentration, and learning. *Panax ginseng* and *Acorus calamus* are found effective in the treatment of memory loss and related symptoms. *Acorus calamus* (Sweet flag) possesses beneficial memory enhancing properties and is used in the treatment of memory impairment. *Acorus calamus* also shows anti-inflammatory, antioxidant, antispasmodic, cardiovascular hypolipidemic, and immunosuppressive.

Other herbs mentioned in their study are: Angelica, Gaduchi, the bark of *Magnolia officinalis*. Lecythidaceae has a high concentration of Lecithin with Choline. Choline is a building block for acetylcholine. Other plants that contain large amount of Lecithin are dandelion flowers, poppy seeds, soybeans, mung beans, horsehound, ginseng, cowpeas, English peas and lentils. Ashwagandha is added here as an antioxidant.

Medicinal plants with a potential to treat Alzheimer and associated symptoms by Anil Kumar Singhal, Vijay Naithani, Om Prakas Bangar Venus Medicine Research Centre, Venus Remedies Ltd., Baddi, H.P, India. National Brain Research Center (NBRC) at Manesar in Haryana, India found that Ashwagandha reversed the AD in mice. Ashwagandha[4] can be effective in the treatment of AD. Suvarna Alladi, Neurologist at the Nizam Institute of Medical Sciences in Hyderabad has been conducting research on how to cure AD. He targeted the liver to remove amyloid plaque from the brain. This is an anti-Amyloid therapy. Kings College, Javalpur of University of Calcutta, reported that basil, turmeric, garlic, ginger, Aloe Vera prevent the breakdown of neurotransmitters; thus, improving memory and concentration in AD. (Tildesley, N.T. Kennedy et al. (2003) Salvia lavandulifolia: may improve word recall in young adults and symptoms of AD.)[5] It enhances memory in healthy young volunteers (*Pharmacology*, *Biochemistry* and *Behavior*, 75(3): 669-74). Large-scale research on complementary medicines for cognition has to be instituted to confirm or deny the claims being made by many who practice alternative and complementary medicine.

Ginkgo biloba, Vitamin E, Brahmi, Gotu Kola and, Acetyl-L-carnitine are used to ward off and treat AD. some of the Australian physicians suggest that complementary medicines should always be included in the medication history of a patient with dementia.[6] A non-judgmental discussion of risks and benefits should be informed by reputable sources of independent information. Possible adverse events should be reported. Patients and their carers should be told never to purchase medicines that lack an Aust L or Aust R number as the quality and safety of these products cannot be assured. Clinical investigations of complementary and alternative medicine are made difficult by factors such as use of complex, individualised treatments and lack of standardisation of herbal medicines.

Pomegranate helps prevent Alzheimer's; it also reduces blood pressure.[7]

Dementia therapies, pharmaceutical or natural, should be used under the supervision of a qualified doctor. FDA has approved the following drugs. They are Donepezil (Aricept); Rivastigmine (Excelon); Galantamine (Razadyne) and Memantine (Namenda).

Alternative drug therapies may be helpful in the treatment of dementia.

Phosphatidylserine (100 mg three times per day).

Antioxidants may protect against the development of dementia. They may even slow the progression of dementia. In some studies, but not all, vitamin E (400-800 IU per day) combined with Aricept was found to slow cognitive decline in people with Alzheimer's disease. Another antioxidant, coenzyme Q10 (10-50 mg three times per day) may supply oxygen to the brain.

Daffodils: Galantamine is present in the leaves and bulbs of daffodils which is effective in the treatment of Mild Cognitive impairment.[8]

B Vitamins: Antioxidants may protect against the development of dementia. Zinc (30-40 mg per day) is often deficient in elderly people, and correcting deficiencies may be helpful to improve memory.

L-arginine: This amino acid has some evidence to suggest that it may help in vascular dementia by increasing blood flow to the brain. The dose used was 1.6 gm each day for three months. Arginine may worsen herpes infections and can interfere with some medications, including Viagra and anti-hypertension medicines. Essential fatty acids such as those found in alpha linolenic acid (ALA), borage oil, and evening primrose oil are used by some people. These omega-3 fatty acids may help reduce the risk of Alzheimer's disease. Dietary changes include eating fewer animal fats and more fish.

Ginkgo (Ginkgo biloba, *Huperzia serrata*), may improve memory in both vascular and Alzheimer's dementia, according to several studies in China.

Lemon balm (*Melissa officinalis*) and Bacopa (*Bacopa monnieri*) leaf extract, called Brahmi, are used in Ayurvedic or Indian medicine to improve brain function and learning.

Lavender may be effective in terms of alleviating agitation associated with dementia. Lavender is not used internally but rather as an aromatherapy agent.

Alternative therapies may help treat dementia. Dementia therapies, pharmaceutical or natural, should be used under the supervision of a qualified doctor.

A growing number of herbal remedies, and dietary supplements to delay or prevent Alzheimer's disease and related dementias have been reported by researchers and others. Claims about the safety and effectiveness of these products, however, are based largely on testimonials, tradition and a rather small body of scientific research. The rigorous scientific research required by the U.S. Food and Drug Administration (FDA) for the approval of a prescription drug is not required by law.

FDA is concerned about these medical foods because the effectiveness and purity of them are unknown. Dietary supplements can have serious interactions with prescribed medications. No one should take a supplement without first consulting a physician.

Alternative treatments that have come to the notice of FDA are the following:[9-11]

- Caprylic acid and coconut oil
- Coenzyme Q10
- Coral calcium
- Ginkgo biloba
- Huperzine A

- Omega-3 fatty acids
- Phosphatidylserine
- Tramiprosate

Caprylic Acid (Coconut Oil)

This is clinically tested as Ketasyn [AC-1202] and marketed as a "medical food" (called Axona®) and coconut oil. The theory behind Axona is that the ketone bodies derived from caprylic acid may provide an alternative energy source for brain cells. The company did not want to test this further at phase 111 required by FDA.

Coenzyme Q10, or Ubiquinone

This is an antioxidant that occurs naturally in the body and is needed for normal cell functions. This compound has not been studied for its effectiveness in treating Alzheimer's. Safe dosage administration of coenzyme Q10 is not known.

Coral Calcium

"Coral" calcium supplements have been heavily marketed as a cure for Alzheimer's disease, cancer and other serious illnesses.

Ginkgo Biloba

Ginkgo biloba is a plant extract containing several compounds that may have positive effects on brain cells. Ginkgo biloba is thought to have both antioxidant and anti-inflammatory properties, to protect cell membranes and to regulate neurotransmitter function. Ginkgo has been used for centuries in traditional Chinese medicine and currently is being used in Europe to alleviate cognitive symptoms associated with a number of neurological conditions. The National Institutes of Health, USA reported that ginkgo was no better than a placebo.

Huperzine A (pronounced HOOP-ur-zeen)

This is a moss extract that has been used in traditional Chinese medicine for centuries. It has properties similar to those of cholinesterase inhibitors one class of FDA approved Alzheimer's medications. As a result, it is promoted as a treatment for Alzheimer's disease. Participants taking Huperzine-A experienced no greater benefit than those taking a placebo. Taking these unregulated preparations could increase the risks of serious side-effects, especially if used in combination with FDA approved Alzheimer's drugs.

Omega-3s are a type of polyunsaturated fatty acid (PUFA). Research has linked high intake of omega-3s to a possible reduction in risk of dementia and cognitive decline. The FDA recommends taking no more than a combined total of three grams of DHA or EPA.

Phosphatidylserine

Phosphatidylserine (pronounced FOS-fuh-TIE-dil-sair-een) is a kind of lipid, or fat that is the primary component of the membranes that surround nerve cells.... The treatment with phosphatidylserine is to protect cells from degenerating. Supplements containing phosphatidylserine are now derived from soy extracts. U.S. Food and Drug Administration (FDA) concludes that there is little scientific evidence supporting the claim that it may reduce the risk of dementia in elderly population.

Tramiprosate (clinically tested as Alzhemed, marketed as a "medical food" called ViviMind™)

Tramiprosate is a modified form of taurine, an amino acid found naturally in seaweed. Amino acids are the chemical building blocks of proteins. Tramiprosate was tested in a large Phase 3 clinical study as a possible Alzheimer's treatment. Analysis of the Phase 3 trial data was initially inconclusive for a variety of reasons. Investigators tried to work with the FDA to obtain clearer results, but the manufacturer decided not to develop Tramiprosate.

Alternative Treatments for Alzheimer's Disease (Investor center).[12]

By Leo Sun, The Motley Fool (Nov. 24, 2013).

Blood Pressure Treatments

A recent study conducted at Johns Hopkins University revealed that blood pressure medications known as ACE inhibitors reduced the risk of Alzheimer's disease by 50 per cent, based on data gathered from a group of 2,200 adults between 75 and 96 years of age.

Rheumatoid arthritis treatment drugs could also be viable treatments for Alzheimer's disease.

Diabetes treatments: The researchers believe that Victoza could possibly reverse memory loss in late-stage Alzheimer's disease and prevent the buildup of Beta-amyloid plaques.

Several alternative methods are suggested to treat Alzheimer's.[13-16]

Ergoloid Mesylates[17] are derived from Rye fungus. The remedy has been used already in Europe. Early research has shown positive results but more testing is necessary. Ergoloid mesylates can be given in liquid or pill form. They are neuroprotective antioxidants and increase blood flow to the brain. Further studies are needed to confirm their benefits for the brain.

Melissa officinalis is commonly known as lemon balm.[18] The Tehran University of Medical Sciences study, found that *Melissa officinalis* extract is valuable in the management of patients with Alzheimer's disease. Other studies show that Lemon balm improves cognition, mood, and decreases stress in patients.

In a study conducted by the Tehran University of Medical Sciences and Institute of Medicinal Plants, *Salvia officinalis* improved the cognitive function with no side-effects in patients. Salvia officinalis has been used in medicine for centuries.

Zizyphus Spinosa

Zizyphus is derived from the fruit of the *Zizyphus jujuba*.

Plant. Zizyphus has been used by traditional Chinese medical practitioners to treat memory problems by nourishing the heart, helping the liver, and calming the mind. It is mainly used for sleep disturbances. Zizyphus treats weakness, fatigue, and distress due to weakness, which causes insomnia (Subhuti Dharmananda, Ph.D., Director, Institute for Traditional Medicine, Portland, Oregon)[19].

Several alternative methods are suggested to treat Alzheimer's.[20] Yi Gan San is a mixture of seven herbs. Ba Wei Di Huang Wan or BDW is a mixture of eight herbs. In a Brazilian medical study, these two herbal formulas were found to be beneficial in treating Alzheimer's disease. Both of these herbal mixtures improve cognition. Yi Gan San in addition is a calming sedative. In several studies, the Chinese herbs *Lycoris radiata*, *Macleaya cordata*, or boluohui; *Coptis chinenses*, or huanglian; and *Securinega suffruticosa*, or yiyiqiu, were found to be effective in treating patients suffering from mild to moderate Alzheimer's disease. They improve cognitive abilities. These herbs have long been used in traditional Chinese and Ayurvedic medicines to treat many different symptoms.

Vitamin D[21-25] is recommended to improve cognitive abilities.

In several scientific studies and clinical trials, vitamin D has been found to be beneficial for the brain. It is able to control pro-inflammatory cytokine, a contributor to cognitive dysfunction. Lack of proper nutrition can contribute to neurodegenerative Alzheimer's disease. In this latest systematic review of the literature, people with Alzheimer's disease (AD) had lower concentrations of vitamin D than those without AD, and better cognitive test results were linked to higher vitamin D concentrations (Balion, C. Griffith L.E. et al., 2012).

Brain relies on vitamin D receptors for protection against the things that can damage it, including the development of the plaques and tangles that form in AD. Both vitamin D and curcumin have been shown to help fight Alzheimer's disease independently. It may be more effective if both of these are administered together.

Only a few foods in nature contain vitamin D. The flesh of fatty fish (such as salmon, tuna, and mackerel) and fish liver oils are among the best sources. Small amounts of vitamin D are found in beef liver, cheese, and egg yolks.

Scandinavian study revealed that vitamin D3 together with curcumin may help stimulate your immune system to clear your brain of amyloid beta, thereby helping to prevent Alzheimer's.

Ergoloid Mesylates:[26] The medication is used to treat problems with mood, memory, concentration or behaviour in the elderly. It is believed to increase blood flow to the brain. It is a combination of three ergot alkaloids. Adhere to the physician's directions in taking this medicine. The medication has side-effects like dizziness, drowsiness, flushing, loss of appetite or stomach upset may occur.

This traditional medicinal herb improved long-term memory impairment in medical trials with mice.[27] Its active principal, 1,2,3,4,6-penta-O-galloyl-beta-D-glucopyranose, has also been found in another herb, *Paeonia suffruticosa*. In another study, it was proved to have potent anti-aggregation effects on Alzheimer's Amyloid beta proteins U.S. Department of Agriculture, Agricultural Research Service, 2011 (USDA National Nutrient Database for Standard Reference. Nutrient Data Laboratory Home Page).

Citrus oil and orange oil: Boost your memory with essential oils. Citrus oils energies the mind. Orange and grapefruits oils are helpful for memory. Lemon oil in particular is a great stress reliever, and helps with concentration. These oils can be used alone or in combination to help boost memory.

Za'atar is associated with ritual purity as mentioned in Hebrew Bible. It has been found in the tomb of Tutankhamun and used as a royal perfume. It is used in cuisines in the Middle East. It makes the mind and body strong. Children are encouraged to eat Za'atar Sandwich for breakfast before an exam or before school. Maimonides, rabbi and physician prescribed Za'atar for its health advancing properties. Za'atar is prepared with thyme, oregano, marjoram and sesame seeds. Another preparation is by adding savory, cumin, coriander or fennel seed.

Shalihan who writes on herbs and usage have mentioned the following.[28] Some physicians knowledgeable on herbs have criticised him. He recommends alpha lipoic acid, acai, goji, mangosteen and so on. He further states that a high concentration of Silica in drinking water may protect against Alzheimer's disease. He also recommends Blue green algae which is a cholinesterase inhibitor.

Herbs to Enhance Cognition and Ward Off Dementia Article Base

Fisher center for Alzheimer's research foundation researched Ginkgo.

The trial, called the Ginkgo Evaluation of Memory, or GEM study, was the largest to date to evaluate the herb. The findings were published in the *Journal of the American Medical Association*.[29]

"Despite early indications that Ginkgo Biloba has antioxidant and other properties that might preserve memory, this trial shows that, in fact, it has no impact on development of dementia and Alzheimer's disease," said lead investigator Dr. Steven T. DeKosky, Director of the University of Pittsburgh.[30-31] Alzheimer's Disease Research Center and Chair of the Department of Neurology at the time the study was conducted.

"Based on the results of this trial, Ginkgo Biloba cannot be recommended for the purpose of preventing dementia," the authors wrote. "These results confirm that randomized trials remain critical to the spectrum of research necessary to develop new therapies."

Spanish Sage (*Salvia lavandulifolia*) may improve word recall in young adults.

Salvia officinalis (common Saga) may improve symptoms of AD.

Sage has been important to herbalists for millennia. It has documented antibiotic and anti-fungal properties. The Romans believed that it had the power to increase lifespan and there's some evidence that it may ward off Alzheimer's. Sage is being investigated as a potential treatment for Alzheimer's disease. MPRC (Maryland Psychiatric Research Center) found that it inhibits an enzyme called acetylcholinesterase (AChE) which breaks down the chemical messenger acetylcholine.

University of Newcastle upon Tyne reports that sage improves memory.[32]

Summary: New research has proved that sage can improve memory, confirming centuries-old theories. British scientists have carried out the first clinical trials with healthy, young adults and found that those who had taken sage oil capsules performed significantly better in a word recall test.

This herb is loaded with very rich source of several B-complex groups of vitamins such as folic acid, thiamine, pyridoxine and riboflavin.

Sage herb, whether fresh or dried, are rich sources of minerals like potassium, zinc, calcium, iron, manganese, copper, and magnesium. Potassium is an important component of cell and body fluids, which helps to control heart rate and blood pressure. Manganese is used by the body as a co-factor for the antioxidant enzyme, superoxide dismutase.

Sage Herb (Salvia officinalis) Nutrition Facts and Health Benefits:[33] Sage is used as a memory enhancer to treat Alzheimer's; it cures inflammation; is an excellent antioxidant. Sage is very versatile to treat many maladies (nutritional facts).[34]

Robin McKie and observer scientists believe that Fasting can help protect against brain diseases.[35]

They claim that giving up almost all food for one or two days a week can counteract impact of Alzheimer's and Parkinson's.

Shilajit[36] is a multimineral found in Himalayan mountains and Caucasus Mountains. It is a powerful anti-aging agent. Shilajit contains 85+ minerals in ionic form and fulvic acid.

With increasing age the cell walls become thick and it becomes increasingly difficult for the minerals and vitamins to be transported deep into the cells. In animals this was beneficial as anti-inflammatory, anti-aging both mental and physical. It is used in Ayurveda. It is not particularly recommended for memory improvement. Shilajit Gold manufactured by Dabur is a powerful rejuvenator.

Shilajit has been used for thousands of years and for as many different health problems. It is listed as a healing agent in ancient Sanskrit writings and is used today in Ayurvedic health practices. Shilajit shows promise in the treatment of Alzheimer's disease, according to a report published in the *International Journal of Alzheimer's Disease* in 2012.[37] According to the report's authors, the fulvic acid found in Shilajit may help block the buildup of tau (a type of protein that forms neurofibrillary tangles, which are a key marker of Alzheimer's disease and other neurodegenerative diseases). However, the report's authors note that a great deal more research is needed to examine Shilajit's effectiveness as an Alzheimer's treatment.

Ashwagandha's botanical name is *Withania somnifera*.[38] Ashwagandha, also called Indian Winter Cherry or Indian Ginseng, is a shrub that is native to India and has been used as a medicinal herb for many centuries.

It improves memory and is known to enhance mental stamina. Ashwagandha, an Indian plant, helps decrease damage caused by stress. It reduces cholesterol and blood sugar levels. Ashwagandha benefits immunity, detoxification and balance; improves memory and concentration; increases the production of oxygen-carrying red blood cells; increases energy; and boosts the brain's production of important neurotransmitters promoting a feeling of well-being; it promotes relaxation and restful sleep.

Health Benefits of Ashwagandha

Scholars at Banaras Hindu University, located in Varanasi, India, have conducted research that has shown that many of the elements of Ashwagandha are antioxidants. The researchers looked at the effects these elements have on the brains of test animals and found that Ashwagandha led to larger amounts of three different natural antioxidants: superoxide dismutase, catalase and glutathione peroxidase. The scholars conclude, "These findings are consistent with the therapeutic use of *W. somnifera* as an Ayurvedic rasayana (health promoter). The antioxidant effect of active principles of *W. somnifera* may explain, at least in part, the reported anti-stress, cognition-facilitating, anti-inflammatory and anti-aging effects produced by them in experimental animals, and in clinical situations." Ashwagandha are therapeutic for thyroid, hair loss, weight loss, fights stress, strengthens immunity" (Ashwagandha Benefits and Side Effects Natural HerbsGuide.com (naturalherbsguide.com/ashwagandha.html)).[39]

Introduction to Ashwagandha

Ashwagandha has been used as a herbal remedy for hundreds of years. It has many applications, and has been used by native Americans and Africans. Because Ashwagandha has traditionally been used to treat various diseases associated with nerve tissue damage related to the destructive molecules known as free radicals, some researchers have speculated that the herb may have antioxidant properties. Free-radical damage plays a role in normal aging and in such neurological conditions as Epilepsy, Parkinson's disease and Alzheimer's disease.

Brahmi is known botanically as *Bacopa monnieri*. Brahmi significantly improves the cognitive ability including an accelerated rate of learning and enhanced memory. These effects are optimized after a 12-week period. *Bacopa monnieri* extract was found to reduce beta amyloid deposits in mice. Taken regularly, Brahmi can drastically reduce the chances of developing AD. Brahmi is used for memory enhancement and as Anxiolytic.

Cognitive Improvement: Brahmi significantly improves the speed of visual information processing, learning rate and memory consolidation, thus enhancing learning ability. It increases superoxide dismutase (SOD) levels, catalase (CAT) levels, and glutathione peroxidase (GPX) activities in the brain, which improves cognitive performance.

The following is an abstract of a study reported on the effects of Brahmi on humans. "Seventy-six adults aged between 40 and 65 took part in a double-blind randomized, placebo control study in which various memory functions were tested and levels of anxiety measured. There were three testing sessions: one prior to the trial, one after three months on the trial, and one six weeks after the completion of the trial. The results show a significant effect of Brahmi on a test for the retention of new information. Follow up tests showed that the rate of learning was unaffected, suggesting that Brahmi decreases the rate of forgetting of newly acquired information. Tasks assessing attention, verbal and visual short-term memory and retrieval of experimental knowledge were unaffected. Everyday memory function and anxiety levels were also unaffected."[40-43]

Researchers at the University of Michigan say green tea may help protect your brain against Alzheimer's disease.

Their study found a molecule in green tea blocks the formation of specific proteins in the brain that clump together to cause Alzheimer's. Specifically, researchers found that EGCG in green tea interferes with the development of plaque seen in Alzheimer's and other degenerative brain conditions. The author of the study says that his team will tweak the EGCG molecule and test its ability to prevent plaque development in animals.

The hope is that research could ultimately lead to clinical trials in Alzheimer's patients to refine the use of ECGC to prevent or maybe, treat Alzheimer's Disease.

In the meantime, a few cups of green tea a day may not only keep you sharp, but also reduce your risk of cancer and protect your heart at the same time.

Green tea has been used as a medicine for thousands of years, originating in China but widely used throughout Asia and now in Europe and USA.[44]

Herbs have been used for centuries in cultures all around the world to benefit learning, memory, concentration, and to benefit those with Alzheimer's. One of my patients with Portuguese background was taking several medicines without knowing why she was taking them. She was depressed and confused. She brought a grocery brown bag full of medicines. I telephoned the physician and requested that he removed all those medicines and put her only that was essential for her medical problems if any. She was seeing several physicians. It is the responsibilities of the physicians to check whether the patient is seeing other physicians and why? Can multiple medicines be toxic? Can it lead to memory difficulties? Several psychological factors when treated with multiple medicines can be harmful to the brain. Memory loss can be due to other factors as well. Ayurvedic physicians prescribe medicines based on herbs. These herbs do not interfere or interact with most medications. If changes are not to the satisfaction of the patient, the physician may change the medicines.

Scientists believe that fasting can help protect against brain diseases. They claim that giving up almost all food for one or two days a week can counteract impact of Alzheimer's and Parkinson's.

Robin McKie, science editor *The Observer, Saturday* 18 February 2012 reported 10 incredible health benefits of fasting after his interview with physicians: 1. Fasting promotes detoxification; 2. Fasting rests digestive system; 3. Fasting resolves inflammatory response; 4. Fasting reduces blood sugar; 5. Fasting increases fat breakdown; 6. Fasting corrects high blood pressure; 7. Fasting promotes weight loss; 8. Fasting promotes healthy diet; 9. Fasting boosts immunity 10. Fasting may help to overcome addictions.[45-47]

Fasting has religious significance. Buddhism practices some periods of fasting, usually on full moon days and other holidays. This is a form of freeing the mind and clarify their thoughts. Catholics fast to do penance for sins, and solidarity with the poor; Yom Kippur for atonement for sins and/or special requests made to God. Fasting is commonly practiced on New Moon and during festivals such as Shivaratri, Saraswati puja and Durga puja by Hindus. Women in North India also fast on the day of Karva Chauth. This is beneficial to enhance concentration during meditation or worship; purification for the system; sometimes considered a sacrifice. Muslims fast on Ramadan. Various Muslim customs recommend days and periods of fasting in addition to Ramadan. They refrain from food, drink and in fact lead a puritan and pious life. Some fast on every Monday, some on Thursday. All religions and congregations need the closeness to God. Many religions require fasting as an act of penance, obligation or faith. Over all these practices have health benefits, both physical and mental.[48-49]

The systematic review identified two herbs and herbal formulations with therapeutic effects for the treatment of AD: *Melissa officinalis*, *Salvia officinalis* and Yi-Gan San and BDW (Ba Wei Di Huang Wan). Ginkgo Biloba was identified in a meta-analysis study. All five herbs are useful for cognitive impairment of AD. *M. officinalis* and Yi-Gan San are also useful in agitation, for they have sedative effects. These herbs and formulations have demonstrated good therapeutic effectiveness but these results need to be compared with those of traditional drugs. Further large multicenter studies should be conducted in order to test the cost-effectiveness of these herbs for AD and the impact in the control of cognitive deterioration (*The Use Of Herbal Medicine In Alzheimer's Disease—A Systematic Review* by Leopoldo Luiz dos Santos-Neto et al.).

Best herbs used in Far East to improve memory and Prevent Dementia. Hanbang, the Traditional Korean Medicine (TKM), is an inseparable component of Korean culture both within Korea, and throughout Korean communities worldwide.[50]

Evidence-Linked Herbal Plants of TKM for Memory Improvement:[51] In Korean, "geonmang" is the term referred to as forgetfulness, amnesia or poor memory.

Several plants like *Panax ginseng*, *Poria cocos*, and *Polygala tenuifolia* are described for the treatment of geonmang in the book *Dong-eui-bo-gam*.

Panax Ginseng

Several studies have indicated that the administration of ginseng may improve learning and memory in healthy volunteers.

Polygala Tenuifolia

Polygala tenuifolia (Fam. *Polygalaceae*) is a reputable herb used in TKM for its memory enhancing effects. Radix Polygalae (RP), the root of *P. tenuifolia*, is used in more than half of the most famous Chinese prescriptions for increasing intelligence. Polygalasaponins are the main constituents of this plant responsible for cognitive improvement.

Ginkgo Biloba

Ginkgo has gone through various clinical trials; it was found to be effective in treating patients with AD and multi-infarct dementia, individuals between 55 and 86 years of age with no history of significant neurocognitive dysfunction.

Acorus Gramineus

Consistent with behavioral data, pre-treatment with AGR significantly reduced ischemia-induced cell death in the hippocampal CA1 area. These results demonstrated that AGR have a protective effect against ischemia-induced neuronal loss, as well as learning and memory damage, and that AGR may be useful in the treatment of VD.

Green Tea

Green tea derived from *Camellia sinensis* (Fam. *Theaceae*) is a popular beverage in Asian countries like Korea, China, and Japan. The major polyphenolic constituents in green tea are epigallocatechin-3-gallate.

Molecules. Cognitive impairment was associated with a lower frequency of tea consumption in men, but not women. Total tea consumption (including both green tea and black/oolong tea) improves cognition, memory, executive function, and information processing speed performances.

Angelica the fruits of *Angelica officinalis* was investigated for its effect on anxiety and memory on mice. Male Swiss mice were tested for anxiety and cognition, in the elevated plus maze test (EPM), using two different procedures. It was observed that acute and repeated administration of imperatorin improved different stages of memory processes (both acquisition and consolidation) in a modified EPM test. These results suggest imperatorin to be an interesting therapeutic option in disorders with high anxiety levels and memory impairment. Numerous herbal plants used in TKM are combined in the form of multi-herbal formula that is more effective than individual herbs alone.

Review

Traditional Korean East Asian Medicines and Herbal

Formulations for Cognitive Impairment

Hemant Kumar, Soo-Yeol Song, Sandeep Vasant More et al., Biotechnology, College of Biomedical and Health Sceince, Konkuk University: Angelica the fruits of *Angelica officinalis*. Herb Formulations for Congnitive Impairment.[51]

In-Su Kim and Dong-Kug Choi

Other Herbs used in Far East to improve Memory are: Ginkgo is used as a herbal medicine in some parts of the Far East. Today it is used to improve memory and prevent dementia.

Cathy Wong, N.D. reports that Ginko is beneficial to improve memory in AD. It also enhances blood circulation.

Ginkgo leaves are believed to contain compounds that thin blood and help to improve muscle tone in the walls of blood vessels. This may enhance blood flow.[52]

What are the Safety Concerns?

Constituents in ginkgo leaves may affect blood clotting, so ginkgo leaf extracts shouldn't be used by people with bleeding disorders. People with epilepsy (or anyone with a history of seizures) should avoid ginkgo, because it may increase the frequency of seizures.

Ginkgo leaf products may affect blood sugar levels, so people with diabetes should only use under the supervision of a health care provider (About.com Alternative medicine).

Black Seed: It is called black cumin in India. Recent research on the black seed as an anti-biotic, anti-tumor, anti-inflammatory, anti-histaminic, anti-bacterial, anti-bronchial and immune boosting agent has shown great promise. It is beneficial for memory improvement. Middle Easterners use a teaspoon of Black Seed Oil mixed in 100 mg of boiled mint for at least 15 days to improve memory.

For Sleep Disorder: Use a tablespoon of Black Seed Oil mixed with honey in any hot drink in the evening.[53]

Muscular Pains (General)

Massage the area of pain with Black Seed Oil (Muslim Health Network). The Russians have developed a rich herbal tradition. Some of the herbs grow only in Russia. Herbalism is a highly regarded healing art in Russia. Most medical schools in Russia offer courses in herbal medicine. Treatment of diseases includes pharmaceutical drugs, medicinal herbs and natural therapies such as massage and cupping.

There are many healing plants in Russia. They are the Siberian Ginseng, Rhodiola, and Chaga. Their efficacy was confirmed by the research in the West.

Siberian Ginseng and Korean Ginseng are well-known and widely used adaptogen. It helps reduce stress and improve concentration and memory. It also helps reduce chronic fatigue.

Chaga:[54-56] Siberians call it as "Gift from God", "Mushroom of immortality". The Japanese call it the "Diamond of the Forest". It is a mushroom but as hard as wood. Chaga contains numerous B vitamins, flavonoids, phenols, minerals, and enzymes. It is a great source for pantothenic acid, which vitamin is needed by the adrenal glands as well as digestive organs. It also contains riboflavin and niacin in significant amounts. Chaga contains wild-source minerals and is particularly high in copper, calcium, potassium, manganese, zinc, and iron.

Yet, its most potent ingredient is a special substance known as superoxide dismutase (SOD). This is an enzyme with great potency. Its function is to halt oxidation, especially the toxicity of a free radical known as singlet oxygen. Japanese and Koreans use it regularly. In much of Siberia, Russia, and Eastern Europe it is an essential beverage. While the U.S. Government restricts medical claims, here is what can be said: Chaga has been used as an essential whole food supplement for many years by Russia's long-lived peasants, as well as long-lived villagers of Japan and Korea. These villagers consume it as a daily beverage. They prefer it over common drinks such as tea and coffee. It is often referred to as the "Birch mushroom". Unlike most mushrooms, chaga is a polypore, a fungus with pores instead of gills. It has the appearance of a black, irregular, cracked mass, grows on tree trunks. Siberian chaga contains 215 phytonutrients including 29 polysaccharide or beta glucan derivatives.

Siberian Chaga, unlike the other medicinal mushrooms has an exceptional amount of Betulinic acid and SOD (Super Oxide Dismutase) content. SOD is an extremely potent antioxidant enzyme that fights cellular damage from reactive single oxygen molecules, also known as free radicals. Research suggests that SOD may be the most important enzyme in our body for the control of free radicals, keeping our cell membranes young, supple, and healthy. SOD is one of the most important antioxidants in our body. Chaga has far more SOD than Vitamins C, E and foods like barley grass, seaweed prunes, fish oils, and aromatherapy essential oils.

According to the Korean Nutrition Society, chaga:

1. Increases the defence reactions of an organism
2. Stimulates metabolism in brain cells
3. Has an anti-inflammatory effect when used internally and externally
4. Is an antioxidant
5. Delays the growth of some kinds of tumors
6. Lowers arterial and venous blood pressure

7. Regulates the heart function
8. Decreases sugar level in blood.

According to Russian Medical Academy, chaga:

1. Has positive effect on lung cancer and liver cancer
2. Calms the nervous system
3. Proven medically, it effects positively various stomach diseases and ulcers
4. Stimulates the immune system.

Siberian Chaga is a superior grade medicinal mushroom containing over 215 phytonutrients, including:

Betulinic acid	29 Betaglucans	Saponins
Polysaccharides	SOD antioxidants	Triterpenes
Inotodiols	Organic minerals	Amino acids

Cyrtanthus obliquus grows in birch forests of Russia, Korea, Eastern and Northern Europe, northern areas of the United States, in the North Carolina Mountains and in Canada. Wikipedia.

Rosemary[57]

It has powerful antioxidant properties, and has several phyto-nutrients, and essential acids. This herb improves memory, over all cognitive functions, and helps increase blood flow to the brain. Rosemary prevents the breakdown of acetylcholine, a neurotransmitter that is crucial in both the central and peripheral nervous system. The most important constituents of rosemary are caffeic acid and its derivatives such as rosmarinic acid. Rosmarinic acid has a number of interesting biological activities, for example, it has antiviral, antibacterial, anti-inflammatory and antioxidant properties.

Rich source of antioxidants and anti-inflammatory compounds—these are thought to help boost the immune system and improve blood circulation. Laboratory studies have shown rosemary to be rich in antioxidants, which play an important role in neutralizing harmful particles called free radicals. It improves digestion. It has the potential to enhance memory and concentration. Rosemary contains an ingredient called Carnosi acid that is able to fight off free radical damage in the brain. It prevents brain aging and is protective against breast carcinoma cells. It may be an effective herbal anti-inflammatory and anti-tumor agent. It can promote eye health.

Health Benefits of Korean Ginseng[58]

Healthy Diet Plans Ginseng is an extremely popular herb, particularly in the Far East. The root is considered to be the most valuable part of the plant. The regular use of ginseng tea is believed to improve memory. Ginkgo Balboa: There is growing research that the leaves from this tree (the oldest tree on earth) help to promote better circulation of blood to the brain. It is beneficial to improve concentration, and memory.

Conclusions[59-62]

The Eleuthero root is an adaptogen. Eleuthero has been shown to increase energy and stamina according to University of Iowa research study. It improves immune system. German scientists have reported that it is antiviral. A Polish study showed that it has the potential to reduce LDL ("bad") cholesterol, triglycerides (blood fats) and blood sugar. It also helps prevent internal blood clots that trigger heart attacks and strokes. A Russian animal study shows that it helps normalize heart rhythm (Mother earth Living). Insufficient evidence to rate effectiveness for improving memory, stroke, heart disease, kidney problems, Alzheimer's disease, Attention deficit-hyperactivity disorder (ADHD), chronic fatigue syndrome, high cholesterol, fatigue, fibromyalgia.

Siberian Ginseng has the same chemical properties as Panax Ginseng.

Eleuthero is often called Siberian Ginseng. It improves stamina and enhances immune function, as do Reishi mushrooms.

Siberian Ginseng is generally considered safe when used as directed. However, people with high blood pressure, sleep apnea, narcolepsy, heart disease, mental illness such as mania or schizophrenia, women who are pregnant or breastfeeding, and people with autoimmune diseases such as rheumatoid arthritis or Crohn's disease should not take Siberian Ginseng. Women who have a history of estrogen-sensitive cancers or uterine fibroids should ask their doctor before taking Siberian Ginseng because it may act like estrogen in the body.[63]

The active ingredients in Siberian Ginseng, called eleutherosides, are thought to have health benefits.

Gotu Kola[64]

Many people refer to Gotu kola as brain food and as beneficial for memory function. It is regarded as one of the most spiritual and rejuvenating herbs in Ayurveda and is used to improve meditation. It is an anxiety reducing herbal medicine. It relaxes the muscle.

Rooibos[65]

Rooibos tea protects the brain and nervous system from toxins. Many drink rooibos tea for optimal brain health. 'Rooibos tea has been used by South African communities for centuries and there are many stories of how it was used against certain human ailments. The tea offers protection in various ways. It is a potent antioxidant, which means that it 'mops up' free radicals.

Health Benefits of Rooibos Tea: High mineral content, improves circulation, can protect against Alzheimer's disease. It also induces restful sleep.

Bacopa, also known as Water Hyssop and Brahmi[66]

This herb contains compounds known as bacosides, which helps neurotransmitters to function better. Even back in 1966, there was a study that showed bacopa to be very promising in the area of learning and reasoning. Since then more studies and clinical trials have definitely shown that it is a "brain booster". Bacopa is very promising for prevention of the neurodegenerative diseases. It is an antioxidant which is helpful to reverse cellular damage. Bacopa extract is now being considered as a possible treatment for Alzheimer's and Parkinson's disease. This herb also shows promise as a treatment for attention deficit hyperactivity disorder (ADHD). It can go a long way in keeping your brain and memory sharp.

Study conducted by the Central Drug Institute (CDR) in Lucknow, India concluded that it increases memory; increases mental agility and alertness; increases ability to learn new information and skills; calms the mind, while promoting relaxation; improves academic performance; helps concentration and focus; increases intelligence in healthy adults, while reducing anxiety. Australian study supports these findings.

Brahmi (Bacopa)[67]

Benefits and Uses: Animal study suggested that the herb normalized heart rhythm. *Benefits of Brahmi*: It provides information on Ayurveda, Ayurveda herbs, ayurvedic medicines and herbal remedy.

Ginseng: Ginseng is an Adaptogen. Research shows that ginseng significantly improves athletic performance and the ravages of stress. Japanese researchers showed that the herb reduces the secretion of stress-related hormones. Ginseng also improves immune function. Korean study showed that ginseng reduced blood pressure, a key risk factor for heart disease and stroke. A Russian, the Italian and Danish studies show that the experimental subjects who took Ginseng for nine weeks, did better with their reaction times, abstract thinking, attention, mental arithmetic ability.

The Benefits of Schisandra—Herbal Powerhouse[68-72]

Isolated to the far Eastern part of the world, the Schisandra berry or "five-flavor berry" in China is used for healthy state of homeostasis by aiding adrenal glands. It improves memory and prevents fatigue. Schisandra is used as an "adaptogen" for increasing resistance to disease and stress, increasing energy, and increasing physical performance and endurance.

Schisandra is also used for preventing early aging and increasing lifespan; normalizing blood sugar and blood pressure; and stimulating the immune system and speeding recovery after surgery.

Schisandra chinensis (五味子 in Chinese, pinyin: wǔ wèi zi, literally "five flavor berry") can improve memory and aid digestion. But those who took ginseng showed significant improvement in memory as suggested by a British study. These berries sharpen concentration, improve memory.

Schisandra is considered one of the premium mind tonics of herbalist. It is used to sharpen concentration, improve memory and increase alertness. Yet unlike caffeine and similar stimulants, schisandra does not produce nervousness. In fact, some people consider schisandra mildly "calming," while producing wakefulness and improved focus.

It has even been used in cases of psychosis, with symptoms of hallucination, paranoia and neurosis, with good results. Herbs for Concentration and Memory "Natural News Chinese medicine: Schisandra berry a potent adaptogenic herb Vitamin and Mineral Encyclopedia by Sheldon Saul Hendler MD PhD".

Rhodiola Rosea extract exerts an antifatigue effect that increases mental performance, particularly the ability to concentrate in healthy subjects. Rhodiola significantly reduced symptoms of fatigue and improved attention after four weeks of repeated administration. A 2007 clinical trial from Armenia showed significant effect for a Rhodiola extract in doses of 340-680 mg per day in male and female patients from 18 to 70 years old with mild to moderate depression. No side-effects were demonstrated at these doses. Another study found antidepressant properties.

Rhodiola, also known as Golden Root: Several Russian studies showed that rhodiola helped students perform better under academic pressure, "Rhodiola is the best adaptogen for mind and memory problems" as stated by Hobbs. "I prescribe it for people who complain of fuzzy memory. They've reported good results." Gerbarg, co-author of *The Rhodiola Revolution* (2004), has used Rhodiola to treat more than 150 people suffering from severe depression. In many cases adding Rhodiola to their treatment increased their energy and allowed them to experience more enjoyment in life. Rhodiola also protects the liver, helping the organ recover from exposure to various poisons, according to Russian and Korean animal studies. Some people afflicted with Lyme disease have used it to good advantage.[73]

Curcumin/Turmeric: Turmeric, also known as curcumin is known for its preventive qualities of the degenerative disorders that can increase with age. This isn't just true of the brain, but good for the heart, and helps avoid some cancers as well. Turmeric has some great antioxidant properties to fight Alzheimer's. There have been some great studies done in Singapore where many elderly people were tested. Those that ingested more turmeric over time did much better in the testing of cognitive functions. When the turmeric consumption was increased, these subjects did even better cognitively. The test was done with curries that had turmeric in them. Taking Vitamin D together with curcumin also magnifies its benefits. "Curcumin safeguards the mind against stress and enhances cognitive functioning. It stops the development of growth within the mind as well as slows, otherwise curbs, the start of Alzheimer's and dementia within the aging brain. Overall, eating curcumin is a fantastic way to maintain your mind agile as well as your brain healthy."[74]

Top herbs for memory: Gingko Biloba, Ginseng; Rosemary, Sage Green tea, Rhodiola Rosea, Bacopa, Gotu Kola, Periwinkle, Blueberries.[75]

Ten memory herbs: (1) Ginseng (2) Ginkgo (3) Gotu Kola (4) Green Tea (5) Bacopa (6) Ashwagandha (7) Rhodiola (8) Huperzia (9) Sage (10) Rosemary.[76]

Homeopath assesses all the important factors when determining the most appropriate treatment for each individual. Some of the most common remedies used for dementia are listed below.

- Alumina—for dullness of mind and vagueness
- Argentum nitricum—for dementia with irritability, especially with lack of control over impulses
- Cicuta—for dementia after head injuries, especially with convulsions
- Helleborus—for stupefaction, when a person answers questions slowly and stares vacantly

- Silica—for mental deterioration with anxiety over small details[77]

The belief of some theorists that cannabis combating brain degeneration is debatable.

The prevention and treatment of cognitive decline and dementia: An overview of recent research on experimental treatments by Chittaranjan Andrade and Rajiv Radhakrishnan.[78]

Chinese herb Naohuandan improves cognitive abilities. Shenyin Oral Liquid (SOL) and Modified Wuzi Yanzong Granule were shown to improve MCI. The herbal formulation Memorin (Phyto-Pharma, Kolhapur) improves concentration, memory of verbal and visuomotor tasks. The authors do not convincingly recommend these herbs.

The Ayurvedic Pharmacopoeia of India indicates the use of the dried rhizomes as a brain tonic to strengthen memory and effective in treating psychoneurosis and epilepsy.

Acorus calamus shows neuroprotective effect against stroke and chemically induced neurodegeneration in rats. Specifically, it has protective effect against acrylamide induced neurotoxicity.

Both roots and leaves of *A. calamus* have shown antioxidant, antimicrobial and insecticidal activities. Acorus calamus (Wikipedia, the free encyclopedia).[79]

Acorus Calamus

Acorus calamus has been an item of trade in many cultures for thousands of years. It has been used medicinally for a wide variety of ailments. In Europe, *Acorus calamus* was often added to wine. Herbal medicine, Sweet flag has a very long history of medicinal used in Chinese and Indian herbal traditions. The leaves, stems, and roots are used in various Siddha and Ayurvedic medicines. It is widely employed in modern herbal medicine as its sedative, laxative, diuretic, and carminative properties. It is used in Ayurveda to counter the side effects of all hallucinogens.

Acorus calamus shows neuroprotective effect against stroke and chemically induced neurodegeneration in rats. Specifically, it has protective effect against acrylamide induced neurotoxicity both roots and leaves of *A. calamus* have shown antioxidant, antimicrobial and insecticidal activities. Calamus root has been used to treat a number of ailments. It also has sedative, laxative, and diuretic properties, counteract the side effects of Hallucinogens. Users of Calamus root report: Alertness, feeling more energetic, feeling less anxiety, relief from sore throat, relief from headaches, a decrease in the side effects of Hallucinogens. Unlike many herbs used for their healing and spiritual properties. Calamus root has a very agreeable taste. It has been proved for its analgesic and anticonvulsant, hepatoprotective, antioxidant, antimutagenic, sedative and hypothermic effects. Good in clearing speech to the children and useful in schizophrenic psychosis. Anticonvulsant activity of raw and classically processed Vacha (*Acorus calamus Linn.*) rhizomes was found.

The rhizome of Vacha (*Acorus calamus*) has been used in Ayurvedic medicine for the treatment of various ailments, such as epilepsy, headache, eye disorders, insomnia, loss of memory, etc. Previous studies demonstrated that Vacha rhizome is having significant anticonvulsant activity.

The results obtained from the present study clearly confirmed the anticonvulsant activity of raw Vacha and subjecting to classical Shodhana procedure did not alter the efficacy of Vacha rhizomes instead it enhanced the activity profile of the Vacha. (Savitha, D. Bhat, B.K. Ashok, R.N. Acharya, and B. Ravishankar Ayu. 2012 Jan-Mar; 33(1): 119-122. PMCID: PMC3456849: Vacha (*Acorus calamus*) effective in treating psychoneurosis and epilepsy).

Neurologists at Murdock St, Wichita, KS, Conducted research on several herbs that enhance Memory and Mental Function. They chose Bacopa Monniera (Brahmi), Ginkgo, Ginseng, and Phosphatidylserine Carnitine as principal natural treatments.[80] They combined two herbs like Ginseng and Ginkgo; vinpocetine and ginkgo. Some improvement was shown in cognitive abilities. It is suggested that combination of phosphatidylserine and ginkgo may be more beneficial. On the other hand, brahmi with ginkgo did not improve cognitive abilities.

Phosphatidylserine: Memory improved amongst those who suffered from severe memory loss. Ginseng with ginkgo showed inconsistent results in memory functions. Their study suggests that Huperzine A, may be helpful for healthy people.

Natural Health News and holistic healing. Top 10 Herbs for Memory.[81]

Gingko Biloba: It aids memory, blood circulation and is good for Alzheimer's. Scientific studies discovered gingko's potency to aid memory and thinking of those with Alzheimer's or vascular dementia by protecting nerve cells damaged by these disorders to improve learning, daily activities, social behavior and reduce feelings of depression.

Ginseng: Good for memory impairment. Ginseng was shown to activate neurotransmitter activities that promote memory enhancement.

Rosemary: It improves memory.

Sage: Experiments have shown that sage boosting the same brain chemicals that drop when one is afflicted by Alzheimer's.

When scientists from the Universities of Newcastle and Northumbria treated animals with the extracts from sage showed better spatial learning abilities and studies suggest that this plant can protect the hippocampus from age-related decline.

Rhodioa Rosea enhanced memory and concentration. One study revealed that intake of rhodiola regularly can increase one's memorization abilities (Examine.com).

Bicopa: In ayurvedic medicine, Bicopa has been used since old times to enhance learning, concentration and memory. (Australian study). After 12 weeks, researchers found out that there has been a significant improvement on the subjects' verbal learning abilities, speed of information processing and memory. Today, Bicopa is widely used as a treatment for memory problems.

Gotukola enhanced memory and concentration. According to studies, Gotukola contains certain substances that increase brain power and improves blood circulation to the brain which results to better memory, concentration, intelligence, and attention span.

Periwinkle: A few researchers claim that periwinkle works like Ginkgo Biloba in enhancing memory. Its vinpocetine content acts as a powerful scavenger of free radicals. This chemical prevents any damages to the blood vessels thereby preventing dementia and senility.

Blueberries: In a study conducted at Harvard University, intake of blueberries helps in boosting brain power. Also, it has been found to aid in staving off cognitive decline and in preventing memory loss that normally comes with aging.

AYURVEDIC MANAGEMENT OF SELECT GERIATRIC DISEASE[82]

Management approaches

a. Prevention

1. Use of special variety of rice, mudga (phaseolus bean), dhiroa, godugdha (freshly milked cow's milk), leaves of brahmi (Indian pennywort), (a variety of amaranth) and vāstuka (a variety of chenopodium), leaf and fruit of papola (a variety of small cucumber), (a variety of pumpkin gourd) and (grape fruit).
2. Use of green vegetables and yellow fruits (apple, papaya, guava, mango, banana, etc.).
3. To live an active life mentally and physically.
4. Consume low fat and rich antioxidant rich foods.
5. Correction of hypertension and diabetes mellitus.
6. Avoid incompatible and hot spicy food articles.
7. Avoid suppression of natural urges like sleep, hunger and thirst.

Drug therapy: SINGLE DRUGS are available.

"COMPOUND FORMULATIONS Drug Dosage (per dose) MOA$/Vehicle Duration"

Brahmi vati: 250-500 mg Honey
15 days

SivaGutika!: 15 days	6 gm	Milk
Cyavanaprasavaleha 15 days	15-30 gm	Milk
Sarpagandhidi 15 days	250 mg	Butter Milk
Manasa mitra vataka 15 days	125 mg	Milk
Kalyana ghrta 15 days	6 gm	Luke warm water

Herbal combination of Shilajit, Ashwagandha (*Withania somnifera*) and Brahmi (*Bacopa monnieri*) are supplements that could help in protecting against brain degenerative diseases and dementia like Alzheimer's disease. Ayurvedic treatments for neurological disorders will aim to rectify the vata imbalance and bring the vata dosha in harmony with pita and kapha dosha so as to eliminate every type of disease in an individual.[83]

Homeopathy[84]

Homeopathy is an ancient treatment.

Unani[85]

Unani is an ancient method of therapy originated in India. Some say that Unani has its origin in ancient Greece. Unani treatment is believed to be founded by Hakim Ibn Sina. Unani practitioner diagnoses health problems by analysing temperament and evaluating the humors. Blood, phlegm, black bile and yellow bile are known as humors. Humors are believed to have capabilities of changing the metabolism of a person.

Siddha[86]

The treatment of Siddha medicine is aimed at keeping the three humors in equilibrium and maintenance of seven elements. Physician recommends proper diet and medicine. Thiruvalluvar explains four requisites for successful treatment. They are the patient, the attendant, physician and medicine. When the physician is well-qualified and the other agents possess the necessary qualities, even severe diseases can be cured easily, according to these concepts.

This concept of the siddha medicine is termed as pathiyam and apathiyam, which is essentially a list of "do's and don'ts". Both Ayurvedic treatment and Siddha are very strict and ritualistic about dos and don'ts.

While Ayurveda was practiced by the 'upper caste' physicians, for the welfare of 'upper caste' people, Siddha was not confined to any caste system and the physicians treated every patient. Ayurvedha, due to its Vedic roots, patronized the Varna system or the caste system, whereas the Siddha system did not believe in the caste system and hence was democratic and progressive.

Other Practices: Mind and Body Practices[87]

These techniques can be used for both treatment and prevention of Alzheimer's.

These mind and body practices are good for overall health and thus good for the brain as well. The following practices may keep brain healthy and ward off Alzheimer's. The practices are recommended for Alzheimer's patients as well.

Mind and body practices include a large and diverse group of procedures or techniques administered or taught by a trained practitioner or teacher.

Habilitation therapy (HT) focuses on ADs remaining overall abilities. Positive emotional state, autonomy, better self-image and morale are the outcome of HT. In addition, all forms of activities will keep ADIs peaceful, physically and mentally happy. This status is helpful for people around them especially care-givers.

Massage therapy includes many different techniques in which practitioners manually manipulate the soft tissues of the body.

Most meditation techniques such as mindfulness meditation or transcendental meditation, involve ways in which a person learns to focus attention.

Movement therapies include a broad range of Eastern and Western movement-based approaches; examples include Feldenkrais method, Alexander technique, Pilates, Rolfing Structural Integration, and Trager psychophysical integration.

Relaxation techniques such as breathing exercises, guided imagery, and progressive muscle relaxation, are designed to produce the body's natural relaxation response.

Spinal manipulation is practiced by health care professionals such as chiropractors, osteopathic physicians, naturopathic physicians, physical therapists, and some medical doctors. Practitioners perform spinal manipulation by using their hands or a device to apply a controlled force to a joint of the spine. The amount of force applied depends on the form of manipulation used.

Tai chi and *qi gong* are practices from traditional Chinese medicine that combine specific movements or postures, coordinated breathing, and mental focus.

The various styles of yoga used for health purposes typically combine physical postures or movement, breathing techniques, and meditation.

Other examples of mind and body practices include healing touch and hypnotherapy.

National Center for Complementary and Alternative Medicine (NCCAM) September 6, 2013).

Magnet Therapy

Various high and low power magnets are used to treat the patient.

Acupressure

Here mild and specific type of pressure is applied on various acupressure points on the body to stimulate that particular organ. Pressure is applied by tips of fingers or thumb of palms and soles of feet.

Acupuncture

Here instead of pressure the specific acupuncture needle is used to stimulate that particular organ. Both traditional and more modern forms of acupuncture are practiced in the UK. A number of studies have addressed the use of acupuncture for treating chronic low back pain, headache and osteoarthritis of the knee. Several questions have been raised about acupuncture, as to how acupuncture might work such as what happens in the brain during acupuncture treatment.

Aromatherapy

Aromatherapy is based on the theory that essential oils, derived from plants, have beneficial properties. The oils used are concentrated and it is important to use them according to instructions, for example diluting them before applying to the skin. The oils may be applied directly to the skin, often accompanied by massage (see 'Massage', below). The oil is heated on an oil burner to produce a pleasant aroma.

There is some evidence that aromatherapy may be effective in helping people with dementia to relax and that certain oils may have the potential to improve cognition in people with Alzheimer's disease. Research has highlighted the potential benefits of aromatherapy, specifically the use of lemon balm (*Melissa officinalis*) and lavender oil, in the treatment of Alzheimer's disease.

Bright Light Therapy

Sleep disorders and disruptive nocturnal behavior are commonly associated with dementia and present a significant clinical problem.

Bright lights have been found to be beneficial as a treatment for sleep disturbances associated with dementia. In bright light therapy, a person sits in front of a light box that provides about 30 times more light than the average office light, for a set amount of time each day. One small but well-conducted study showed promising effects of bright light therapy on restlessness and disturbed sleep for people with dementia. A more recent study showed that using stronger general lighting in care homes improved cognition in people with dementia, enhanced their sense of night and day, enabled them to sleep better, and reduced levels of depression (Alzheimer's Society). Bright light and Melatonin arrest the progression of dementia, improve sleep and overall improve general behavior.

Reiki

It is based on the concept of energy balance i.e. to cure the energy disturbances which results in development of disease. Reiki is known as oriental medicine; Reiki is a practice of palm healing. Traditional Japanese Reiki and western Reiki are two branches of Reiki. "Do not be angry, do not worry, be grateful, work with diligence, be kind to people." These are the constructing elements of Reiki treatment. The treatment method describes seven major parts of body and their relation with specific points on hand. Reiki uses the instruments of looking, blowing, tapping and touching to heal any disease.

Reflexology

Reflexology is a common practice in modern spas. Reflexology is also known as zone therapy. In this treatment, reflex is created on various body organs with touch at the corresponding points on feet. All the body organs are believed to have connecting or corresponding nerves passing through the feet in reflexology therapy. The feet are divided into 10 parts. Manipulation of these 10 parts is believed to bring in cure from diseases. Again, reflexology is not a proven treatment method.

Pyramid Healing

This treatment claims to provide mental, physical and spiritual wellness. Pyramid therapy tries to use the power associated with pyramid shapes. Different types of pyramids with a master crystal at the extreme top are used in this therapy. A person has to sit in meditative posture within the pyramid to absorb the energy formed within the pyramid. Auroville pyramid temples are famous with foreigners.

Yoga

Yoga has now become a global phenomenon. It is widely recognized for its ability to enhance spititual, emotional and physical health. In Sanskrit, Yoga means union of body, mind and spirit. Yoga taps into our highest potentials. It is practiced for the attainment of perfect equilibrium and harmony; self-healing; removal of negetive thoughts and toxins from the body; enhancement of personal power; self-awareness; reduction of stress and strain by activating the parasympathetic nervous systom and improvement of concentration and cognitive abilities.

Hydrotherapy

In this therapy, only water is used to treat the patient externally or internally with or without additives.

Diet/Nutritional Therapy

In this therapy, food habits are cultivated upon the need of individual. Attention is given to maintain the acid alkaline balance of the body.

Batch Flower Remedy

In this 38 remedies made from flowers are used on the basis of mental state of the patient.

Feng Shui

Feng Shui is another Chinese alternative therapy form which believes the rules of both astronomy and geography will help to generate positive energy and thus sound health and well-being. Feng Shui teachings implement the idea that all the structures we live in have the necessary powers to influence our health and peace. The necessary rearrangement or the presence of certain objects is said to have positive effects in our lives.

Branches of herbal medicine include Western herbal medicine, Chinese traditional medicine, and kampo, a Japanese variant of Chinese medicine. The following herbs may have some effect on symptoms associated with dementia:

- *Choto-san*—Two studies into this kampo (see above) mixture, which contains 11 medicinal plants, have found that it improved a range of symptoms in people with vascular dementia. Further research on this preparation seems justified.

- *Kami-Umtan-To* (*KUT*)—This is another kampo mixture, which contains 13 different plants. A clinical trial found a slower decline in the group of people with Alzheimer's disease given this preparation.
- *Yizhi capsule* (*YZC*)—Initial studies on the use of this Chinese traditional herbal medicine in patients with vascular dementia have reported positive results, although the studies were not of a high standard. Further research into this preparation seems justified, but for now the evidence is inconclusive.
- *Ginkgo biloba extract*—Until recently it was thought that Ginkgo Biloba could be effective at slowing down the progression of dementia and the remedy still has its proponents. However, a study carried out in 2008 found that it has no effect and this was confirmed by reviews of a larger number of small studies. (This is controversial in Western countries.)

Music Therapy

Music can have a powerful effect on a person's state of mind. It is a mood setter. Music has the power to enhance brain functions. Music enhances Reading and literacy skills, Spatial-temporal reasoning, Mathematical abilities, Emotional intelligence and Memory.

Music Therapy usually involves playing music or sounds, such as white noise that the person enjoys for up to 30 minutes in a quiet room. Someone must be present to make sure that the person with dementia is comfortable and happy with the level of sound. This person can encourage the patient to appreciate the music, join in which the rythms or sing along. If ther is a certain time of the day when a person with dementia becomes agitated, music therapy can be scheduled accordingly.

Music appreciation is universal. The choice of music is important. It is used in Reminiscence Thearpy. Western as well as

Indian classical music are beneficial to relax every one including animals and plants. A slower tempo can quiet the mind and relax the muscles. Listening to music can reduce chronic pain. Music is effective for relaxation and stress management. It is beneficial for all human beings. The choice of music is important. It is used in reminiscence therapy. Soft classical Western music is beneficial to relax everyone including animals and plants. (Read more on Music. "Music and Learning" and integrating Music in classroom.)

TENS (transcutaneous electrical nerve stimulation) involves applying a mild electrical current through electrodes stuck to the skin. The treatment can produce a prickling sensation but is not painful. No conclusive data to suggest it is beneficial for dementia. It may be beneficial to reduce pain (Alzheimer's Society-herbal medicine).

Institute of Alternative Medicines and Research:[87] This institute in India provides diploma, degree and post graduate courses in various systems in alternative/complementary/traditional therapies such as acupuncture, naturopathy, yoga therapy, herbal medicine, aromatherapy, traditional Chinese medicine acupressure, Bach flower remedies, chiropractic, kinesiology, etc. through distance learning system. www.altmedschool.com covers United States of America, Canada, United Kingdom, Malaysia, Thailand and Singapore.

Almost all medical schools offer classes in alternative medicine in India. Alternative medicine exists in all cultures to some degree and terms such as traditional medicine, indigenous medicine or folk medicine are used to describe such practices. These medicines date back hundreds of years depending on the country and culture concerned. There are more than 100 systems of alternative medicines still in practice all over the world. Every country, region or area has its own traditional system of health and medical services such as for the Chinese it is acupuncture, for the French magnetic healing; for the Germans Heilpraxis; for the English Herbalism; for India, Ayurveda with Siddha being widely practiced in the southern part of the country; for Japanese Shiatsu and much more.

The most popular forms of alternative medicine are Ayurveda, Homeopathy, Naturopathy, Yoga, Acupuncture, Acupressure, Magneto therapy, Shiatsu, Herbalism, Meditation, Aromatherapy, Bach Flower Remedies, Chromo therapy, Diet therapy, Hydropathy and Reiki. For more information refer to Indian Board of Alternative Medicines.

To quote from Wikipedia the free Encyclopedia[88] Richard Dawkins, an English evolutionary biologist and author, in an essay in his book *A Devil's Chaplain* (2003) (chapter 4.4), has defined alternative medicine as a "set of practices that cannot be tested, refuse to be tested, or consistently fail tests. Another essay in the same book (chapter 1.4) quoted from an article by John Diamond in *The Independent*: "There is really no such thing as alternative medicine, just medicine that works and medicine that doesn't. Dawkins has argued that, if a technique is demonstrated effective in properly performed trials, it ceases to be alternative and simply becomes medicine."

Health and medicine are debated by every adult, physicians, politicians; insurance companies, pharmaceuticals, income tax services, and other professionals over Western and Eastern medicine.

Health is universal. It's a human right, not a privilege. Both Western and alternative medicine have strengths that will grow stronger if practiced with understanding and mutual respect. It helps the patients since they do not have to run around to many different clinics and doctors. The journal of the American Medical Association (JAMA) reported that medical professionals are beginning to integrate western and Eastern (alternative) medicine. JAMA stated that the Medical Schools in USA are now offering courses in alternative medicine. Medical schools of Eastern countries offer alternative medicine as an integral part of medicine.

REFERENCES

Cen Gong: 2014: GABA, Nature Communication, June/14/2014.

Diego Gomez-Nicola, Stephano Suzzi et al. (2014). Temporal dynamics of hippocampal neurogenesis in chronic neurodegeneration: Harvard Health publication, *Journal of Brain*, June 14.

McShane, University of Oxford 2013: G8 Conference on Alzheimer's

Pascual-Leone, Alvero (Jan. 2013). Neuro AD. Harvard Health Publication, Harvard Medical School.

Tanzi Rudi (Jan. 2013): PRT2 Harvard Health Publication, Harvard Medical School.

Yanker Bruce (2014). Harvard Medical School: REST, Huffington Post, 3/19/2014 and Alzheimer's Australia Dementia news March 26 2014.

Alternative Medicine

1. Alzheimer's (www.ayuryogashram.com)
   Kerala Ayurveda treatment (Kerala)
   Welcome to Kerala Ayurveda Limited
2. www.keralaayurveda.biz(Kerala YURVEDA)
3. Anil Kumar Singhal et al. (2012)

   Anil Kumar Singhal, Vijay Naithani, Om Prakash Bangar: Venus Medicine Research Centre, Venus Remedies Ltd., Baddi, H.P., India) Year : 2012 | Volume : 2 | Issue : 2 | Page : 84-91

   Medicinal plants with a potential to treat Alzheimer and associated symptoms.
4. Alzheimer India.Org. (Care of the elderly) National Brain Research Center (NBRC).
5. Tildesley, N.T. Kennedy et al. (2003) enhances Memory in healthy young volunteers. (Pharmacology, Biochemistry and Behavior 75 (3): 669-74.
6. Salvia officinalis (common Sage) may improve symptoms of AD.
7. Pomegranate helps prevent Alzheimer's; it also reduces blood pressure. www.ayurvedictalk.com/pomegranate-helps-prevent-alzheimer's

Drug Therapies

8. Joint Nature Conservation Committee (JNCC) 28/06/2013: Treating Alzheimer's with Daffodils, A natural source for the treatment of Alzheimer's Disease.
9. www.alz.org/aboutad/treatment/alternative.asp\l
10. Alternative Alzheimer Treatments I Health For More
11. www.healthformore.com/alternative-alzheimer-treatments.html\l.
12. Alternative Treatments for Alternative treatments for Alzheimer's.
13. http://www.neurological-recovery-guide.com.
14. Alzheimer's Mayoclinic.org/diseases-conditions/alzheimers-disease/in-depth.
15. Alzheimer'swwa"http://umm.edu/health/medical/altmed/condition/alzheimers-disease" of Maryland Medical Center and umm.edu/health/medical/altmed/condition/alzheimers-disease
16. Treatment. The goals in Am J Alzheimers Dis Other Demen. 2006; 21(2):113-8. Alternative medicine and Alzheimer disease. Neurologist. 2008 Sep; 14(5):299-306.
17. Alternative Treatments for Alzheimer's Disease by Leo Sun, The Motley Fool Nov 24th 2013 10:16AM Updated Nov 24th 2013.
18. Melissa officialis is commonly known as Lemon balm.
    Read more: http//www.livestrong.com/article/301397-chinese herbs –for-Alzheimer's.
19. Journal of medicinal plants research *Journal of Medicinal Plants Research* Vol. 5 (6), pp. 915-921, March 2011.
20. Yi Gan San BS Ba Wei Di Huang Wan. www.Livesrong.com article /301397 Chinese herbs for Alzheimer's.

Vitamin D COUNCIL

21. C. Balion, et al.Vitamin D, cognition, and dementia. A systematic review and meta-analysis. Neurology 2012; 79:1397-1405. Alzheimer's Disease. Alzheimer's Association, 2013. Web. 8 November 2013. www.alz.org.
22. Alzheimer's Disease. Alzheimer's Association, 2013. Web.8 November 2013,www.alz.org.

23. Oudshoorn C, Mattace-Raso FUS, van der Velde N, Colin EM, van der Cammen TJM. Higher serum vitamin D3 levels are associated with better cognitive test performance in patients with Alzheimer's disease. Dementia and Geriatric Cognitive Disorders 2008; 25:539-543 Soni M, Kos K, Lang IA, et al.

24. Vitamin D and cognitive function. *Scandinavian Journal of Clinical and Laboratory Investigation* 2012; 243:79-82.

25. The study revealed that vitamin D3 together with curcumin may help stimulate your immune system to clear your brain of amyloid beta, thereby helping to prevent Alzheimer's.

    Ref: institute of Medicine, Food and Nutrition Board (p. 97) Press 2010.

26. This traditional medicinal herb improved long-term memory impairment in medical trials with mice. Its active principal, 1, 2, 3, 4, 6-penta-O--galloyl-beta-D-glucopyranose, has also been found in another herb, Paeonia suffruticosa. In another study [11] it was proved to have "potent anti-aggregation effects on Alzheimer's Amyloid beta proteins" U.S. Department of Agriculture, Agricultural Research Service. 2011. USDA National Nutrient Database for Standard Reference, Release 24. Nutrient Data Laboratory Home Page, http://www.ars.usda.gov/ba/bhnrc/ndl.

27. www.herbcyclopedia.com/index.php?option=com_zoo&task=item&item_id=

28. www.raysahelian.com/" Sahelian MD. January 20, 2014.

    Herbs to Enhance Cognition and Ward off Dementia Article base.

29. Fisher center for Alzheimer's research foundation.www.ALZinfo.org

30. T. Steven, et al. "Ginkgo biloba for Prevention of Dementia: A Randomized Controlled Trial." *Journal of the American Medical Association*, November 19, 2008, Volume 300, Number 19, pages 2253-2262.

31. Lon S. Schneider, M.D.: "Ginkgo Biloba Extract and Preventing Alzheimer Disease" (editorial). *Journal of the American Medical Association*, November 19, 2008, Volume 300, Number 19, pages 2306-2308.

32. Sage Improves Memory, Study Shows
September 1, 2003; University Of Newcastle Upon Tyne.
Sage herb (*Salvia officinalis*) nutrition facts and health benefits.
33. www.nutrition-and-you.com/sage-herb.html.
34. Umesh Rudrappa - in 56 Google+ circles.
35. Robin McKie, science editor. *The Saturday*, 18 February 2012 .
36. undergroundhealthreporter.com › *Health Conditions* › *Anti-Even More Info:* Shilajit *at* Memory *Forum:* Improve *Your* Memory ...*curezone.org/forums/fm.asp?i=267022*
37. Shilajit shows promise in the treatment of Alzheimer's disease, according to a report published in the *International Journal of Alzheimer's Disease* in 2012. About.com ALTERNATIVE MEDICINE.
38. Ashwagandha Benefits.com.
39. Ashwagandha Benefits and Side Effects | Natural Herbs Guide. com naturalherbsguide.com/ashwagandha.html.
40. Steven Roodenrys Ph.D[1], Dianne Booth MSc[1], Sonia Bulzomi G. Dip.App.Psyc[1], Andrew Phipps G.Dip.App.Psyc[1], Caroline Micallef G.Dip.App.Psyc[1] and Jaclyn Smoker G.Dip. App.Psyc[1]
41. Department of Psychology, University of Wollongong, Wollongong, Australia.
42. Neuropsychopharmacology (2002) 27, 279–281. Doi: 10.1016/ S0893-Can green tea help prevent Alzheimer's Disease? New study.
43. article.wn.com/view/2011/03/16/...preventAlzheimers_Disease_ New_study\. Alzheimer's, cataracts ... All recreational use of these herbs is...
44. Memory Loss | Natural Herbal Homeopathic Ayurvedic Remedies www.healthherbsandnutrition.com/remedies/m/memoryloss.
45. Robin McKie, science editor *The Observer*, Saturday 18 February 2012. Religion and fasting.
46. Seliger, S. & Haines, C.D. (2012). 'Is Fasting Healthy?' Accessed from http://www.webmd.com/diet/features/is_fasting_healthy.

47. Panjwani, M. (2009). '11 Health Benefits of Fasting', Accessed from http://mushpanjwani.com/2009/08/23/11-health-benefits-of-fast.

The use of Herbal Medicine in Alzheimer's disease—A Systematic Review

Leopoldo Luiz dos Santos-Neto,[1] Maria Alice de Vilhena Toledo,[2] Patrícia Medeiros-Souza,[3] and Gustavo Almeida de Souza

48. Evidence Based Complement Alternate Med. 2006 December; 3(4): 441-45.

49. Published online 2006 October 23. doi:10.1093/ecam/nel071

50. Best herbs *used* in Far East to improve memory and Prevent Dementia.

51. Evidence-Linked Herbal Plants of TKM for Memory Improvement:

52. Ginkgo is *used* as a *herbal medicine* in some parts of the *Far East*. Today it is *used* to *improve memory* and *prevent dementia*.

53. Black seed. (www.muslimhealthnetwork.org/ls_black_seed.shtml)

54. Chaga: Siberians call it as "Gift from God" "Mushroom of immortality. Chaga mountain inc. altmedicine.about.com. Alternative Medicine › Supplements. Nutrition Society.

55. Why Use Chaga? - Earthborn Wellness www.earthbornwellness.com/chagause.htm

56. www.chagamountain.com/health-benefits.html

57. Read more: Health Benefits of Rosemary Herb | Rosemary Herb–Health Benefits. http://www.medindia.net/patients/lifestyleandwellness/health-benefits-of-rosemary-herb.htm#ixzz2tYLyuKPf.

58. Health Benefits of Korean Ginseng - Healthy Diet Plans.

www.diethealthclub.com › *Health Food.*

59. Ginkgo Biloba: cognitive impairment and dementia.
Birks J, Grimley EV, Van Dongen M.
Author information Department of Clinical Geratology, University of Oxford.

60. Cochrane Database Syst Rev. 2007; (2):CD003120.

61. Herbs & Herbal Remedies altmedicine.about.com
62. Eleuthero-Health benefits you may not know about.altmedicine. about.com...Herbs and Herbal Remedies. By Cathy Wong
63. *Siberian ginseng* | University of Maryland Medical Centre https://umm.edu/health/.../siberian-ginseng University of Maryland. *www.kcweb.com/herb/gotu.htm*
64. Gotu Kola: www.kcweb.com/herb/gotu.htm
65. Rooibos: Science in Africa march 2005.
66. Read Original Article: http://www.herbslist.net/bacopa.html
67. Brahmi (Bacopa): Benefits and Uses
68. Schizandra berry a potent adaptogenic herb by: Dani Veracity Sunday, July 03, 2005.
69. Learn more: http://www.naturalnews.com/009229_schizandra_schisandra.html#ixzz2u6oJ05O6
70. Vitamin and Mineral Encyclopedia by Sheldon Saul Hendler MD PhD, p. 326.
71. Learn more. http://www.natural schizandra_schisandra.html#ixzz2u6oy4lCd news.com/009229_
72. Read more http://www.ehow.com/list_7463766_herbs-concentration-memory.html#ixzz2tYrCR5wg
73. Rhodiola: (golden root) Read Original Article: http://www.herbslist.net/bacopa.htmlWikipedia, the free encyclopaedia.
74. National college of Singapore. August 8, 2013: Curcumin's benefits for the brain.
75. Sage Herb Shown to Boost Brain Performance, Significantly... Conscious life news.com/sage-herb-shown-boost-brain-performance-significantly-impr... Aug 27, 2013... Recent studies on sage indicate that the herb can improve memory and even possibly prevent Alzheimer's disease.
76. Ten memory Herbs- progressive Health.com
77. Silica—for mental deterioration with anxiety over small details Source: Dementia | University of Maryland Medical Center http://umm.edu/health/medical/altmed/condition/dementia#ixzz2sQ4kumWE

78. Chittaranjan Andrade and Rajiv Radhakrishnan Indian J Psychiatry. (2009 Jan-Mar): The prevention of mild cognitive impairment in Alzheimer's disease.

79. https://en.wikipedia.org/wiki/Acorus_Calamus: Acorus Calamus is neuroprotective against stroke and neurotoxicity,epilepsy.

    - Acorus calamus shows neuroprotective effect against stroke and chemically induced neurodegeneration in rats. Specifically, it has protective effect against acrylamide induced neurotoxicity
    - Both roots and leaves of A. Calamus have shown antioxidant, antimicrobial and insecticidal activities Acorus calamus, From Wikipedia, the free encyclopedia

80. A WesleyCare Clinic. Enhancing Memory and Mental Function. EBESCO Enhancing and Memory Function. (Continuous revision) Phosphatidylserine combined with Ginko improved memory amongst those suffered from severe memory loss.

81. www.undergroundhealth.com/top-10-herbs-for-memory. October 3, 2013

82. ccras.nic.in/.../4.% 20Ayurvedic_Management_of_Select_Geriatric_Disease.

83. Institute of Medicine, Food and Nutrition Board. USDA (United States Drug Administration)

84. HOMEOPATHY:

    Silica—for mental deterioration with anxiety over small details. Source: Dementia University of Maryland Medical Center. http://umm.edu/health/medical/altmed/condition/dementia#ixzz2sQ4kum WE85)

85. Unani

86. Sidha

87. Other alternative treatments:www.aaltmedschool.com

8

Caregiving

In USA, 80 per cent of care is provided to AD patients by family members. In India family members will hardly think of placing the AD patient in a nursing home because of familial, societal and cultural beliefs. It is implicit within the family culture that older people will be taken care of by their children in the patient's home where the patient belongs. "Honor your parents and respect them" is within the consciousness of the Indian children. Nursing home is not a sociological construct within the context of Indian families. Most of the people I talked to informed me that it is unthinkable to admit their parents in a nursing home or an assisted living or elder care while the AD patient has a home and family to take care of her/him. My cook told me "They took care of us when we needed them and now it is our turn to take care of them." Traditionally, it is built into the family system that children take care of their parents when they are old or disabled. There is no debate on this.

However, the family as a system with built-in cultural values is gradually changing due to socio-economic factors and impact of foreign values. The professional adults in the family, who take up lucrative jobs in foreign countries, are compelled to think in alternate ways of taking care of their aged and AD parents. Traditionally, it is incumbent upon daughters and daughters-in-law to take care of the parents. The role of the sons is to take care of them financially and take overall responsibilities for them.

Daytime care is easily available for ADs in India from the family members, maids, cooks and paid caregivers. Caring for a patient with AD is often very difficult. Family members and other unpaid caregivers experience high levels of physiological and psychological stress, anxiety, and despondency. They may express mixed emotional reactions to stressful situations and then feel guilty. The employed relatives find that the responsibility of taking care of their ailing parents is an additional responsibility. Only a few are attuned to take care of older people. Dutiful children relegate their duties as a matter of fact, giving up their social life. In India, the social life is limited to extended family mostly unlike in US. Traditionally, the oldest son and his wife are expected to take care of the parents. The oldest son has an important role to play in management of property, family home, wealth and assets. His wife may share these responsibilities. People adhere to traditional cultural values that are prescribed by Vedas, scriptures and myths. "It is a way of life." In India, extended family is a society by itself, although currently this system is showing some variations. Daughters even though they may have their own family to take care of often opt out to take care of their parents. They do not want to leave their parents to the mercy of hired caregiving people for fear that the parents may be physically and mentally abused.

India is a multi-cultural, multi-religious society. India's architecture, languages, religions, beliefs, veritable dances, music from classical to folk songs, attire, jewelry, cuisines and customs that differ from place to place from state to state are unique and are very different from Western culture.

The Golden Rule

Golden Rule is an ethical statement which is found in many religions and philosophies. It is also called the ethics of reciprocity. The following religious faiths are taken from Wikipedia.

BUDDHISM — "Just as I am so are they, just as they are so am I," he should neither kill nor cause others to kill (Sutta Nipata 705)

One who, while himself seeking happiness oppresses with violence other beings who also desire happiness, will not attain happiness hereafter.

CONFUCIANISM "What you do not wish for yourself, do not do to others."

EXISTENTIALISM What we choose is always the better; and nothing can be better for us unless it is better for all. (Jean).

HINDUISM One should never do that to another which one regards as injurious to one's own self. This, in brief, is the rule of dharma. Other behavior is due to selfish desires.

Brihaspati, Mahabharata (Anusasana Parva, Section CXIII, Verse 8.)

Also, if the entire "Dharma" (spiritual and moral laws) can be said in a few words, then it is—that which is unfavorable to us, do not do that to others. (Padmapuraana, Shrushti 19/357-58)

CHRISTIANITY According to Simon Blackburn, although the Golden Rule "can be found in some form in almost every ethical tradition", the rule is "sometimes claimed by Christianity as its own". The Golden Rule has been attributed to Jesus of Nazareth: "Therefore all things whatsoever would that men should do to you, do ye even so to them" (Matthew 7:12, see also Luke The common English phrasing is "Do unto others as you would have them do unto you."

HUMANISM "Do not treat people in a way you would not wish to be treated yourself". Empathy is at the root of kindness, compassion, understanding and respect.

According to Marc H. Bornstein and William E. Paden, the Golden Rule is arguably the most essential basis for the modern concept of human rights, in which each individual has a right to just treatment, and a reciprocal responsibility to ensure justice for others.

ISLAM Not one of you is a believer until he loves for his brother what he loves for himself (Islam, Forty Hadith of an-Nawawi 13). Prophet in Qur'an said: "As you would have people do to you, do to them; and what you dislike to be done to you, don't do to them. By Kitab unnah Woe to those...who, when they have to receive by measure from men, they demand exact full measure, but when they have to give by measure or weight to men, give less than due" Qur'an (Surah 83, "The Dealers in Fraud," vv. 1-4). "Orphans and the needy, give them something and speak kindly to them. And those who are concerned about the welfare of their own children after their death, should have fear of God [Treat other people's Orphans justly] and guide them properly" Qur'an (4, "The Women," vv. 8-9).

PLATONIM The Golden Rule appears to be present in at least one of Plato's dialogues: One should never do wrong in return, nor mistreat any man, no matter how one has been mistreated by him. "Plato's Socrates" (Crito, 49c) (c. 469 BC-399 BC)

JAINISM In Jainism, the Golden Rule is firmly embedded in its entire philosophy and can be seen in its clearest form in the doctrines of Ahimsa and Karma.

The following quotation from the Acaranga Sutra sums up the philosophy of Jainism: "Nothing which breathes, which exists, which lives, or which has essence or potential of life, should not be destroyed or ruled over, or subjugated, or harmed, or denied of its essence or potential. "Just as sorrow or pain is not desirable to you, so it is to all which breathe, exist, live or have any essence of life. To you and all, it is undesirable, and painful, and repugnant." (Jainism, Sutrakritanga 1.11.33)

"In happiness and suffering, in joy and grief, we should regard all creatures as we regard our own self." "A man should wander about treating all creatures as he himself would be treated"(Sutrakritanga 1.11.33). "One should treat all beings as he himself would be treated." (Agamas Sutrakritanga 1.10.13)

JUDAISM The Jewish Publication Society's edition of Leviticus: Thou shalt not take vengeance, nor bear any grudge against the children of thy people, but thou shalt love thy neighbor as thyself: I am the LORD. What is hateful to you, do not do to your fellowman. This is the entire Law; all the rest is commentary. (Talmud, Shabbat 3id)

SIKHISM See also: *Sikhism and Karma*. Whom should I espise, since the one Lord made us all? (p. 1237, Var Sarang, Guru Granth Sahib, tr. Patwant Singh)

Sikhism "As thou deemest thyself, so deem others."

TAOISM Regard your neighbor's gain and your neighbour's loss as your own loss. (Tai Shang Kian Yin P'ien)

All religions respect fellow beings irrespective of their faith. One concept that runs through all these religions is the concept of empathy. It represents a broad range of emotional stages such as caring for other people and having a desire to help them. Compassion and sympathy are embedded in it. To get into the very existence of another person is a sophisticated imaginative process. People can be trained to be sympathetic and empathetic with others who are not privileged.

Psychologists and neuroscientists are interpreting the empathy from a neurological point of view. Measures of empathy show that mirror neurons are activated during arousal of sympathetic responses and prolonged activation show increased probability to help others. Research in this area shows the many vicissitudes of emotions and empathy.

There are many retirement homes for older people all over India. Some of these homes are run very efficiently taking care of all the needs of the older patients. Home atmosphere is maintained in these facilities, so that they feel very secure physically, emotionally and socially. However, much we may justify this situation, the AD patients will have a yearning for their own home with all the comforts and security of the home. Home has a history and life of its own. Memories associated with the home may stay alive because of remembrance of events associated with the home, and multiple emotions attached to it. A person's very existence comes alive in one's own home. Some communities in India worship their ancestors and the walls of the home are adorned with the photographs of the departed ancestors. They start the day by doing Puja (prayer) to the departed souls.

Living in one's own home affords physical, emotional, and social well-being, with friends and relatives in the neighborhood who could be contacted at any time of the day or night. Above all "home is where the heart is; the comfort space". The surroundings are familiar. The hospitals, physicians, the helpers at home like the cook, the maids, valet, watchman, the Dhobi (one who cleans the clothes and iron), the gardener, shop-keepers, the pharmacy, the butcher, the barber and the baker, milkman, newspaperman, sweeper, the flower seller, neighbors and so on over the years have become extensions of one's family. Leaving one's own home to go to a strange place means leaving all those people that they see every day and whose happiness and tragedies become their own. In extended families, there will be many inconveniences and likes and dislikes, but each person can find their own physical psychological spaces. For poor people old age is only an existence and they depend on the mercy of the community, social and religious organizations.

One analyst observed that "The breakdown of the family commenced when the Maharajas, India's regional kings, were deposed. Until then, these monarchs and their families regulated society and kept the joint and extended family structure intact." Indian culture and ethics prescribe that older people should not be neglected. Today some seniors are left in the lurch because of the transfer of estates and assets to their children. In the West, this transaction takes place after death through a legal will. In India it has been common to legally transfer such properties and accounts long before death. When performed ethically, this practice frees the elder of the burden of property and money management. It is an unsaid/unwritten value system that children will take care of old parents. But in an inhuman twist of fate, a retired Indian administrative officer has been forced to spend the last few days of his life in an old age home. Indignant, he explained that he had transferred his assets to his son. His wife was allowed to stay at home as a maid. Psychologically, socially and from family point of view this must have been devastating.

Overall, children and relatives can be trusted with their lives compared to strangers in a nursing home/retirement homes.

Little sisters of the poor in Chennai take care of a few ADIs who have no relatives. They are provided with all the amenities that are expected and protected from all the negative forces that would harm them physically and emotionally. The ADIs are really provided a home with all the best that the sisters can provide for them. The two Holy Sisters from Belgium who are getting older are very caring and understanding of the needs of the ADIs. On the other hand, there are places where ADIs are only given shelter and provided with the basic needs. These ADIs just exist.

Care Giving Tasks for moderate AD patients:

Activities of Daily Living (ADLs): Encourage ADIs to have a specific time to wake up in the morning and adhere to activities of the day. As far as possible encourage the ADIs to follow the routine that the person practiced prior to becoming a patient. Behaviors can be modified through conditioning.

Hygiene is very important for the patient and for others who are around the ADIs. It is incumbent upon the CG to maintain the hygiene of the patient. The CG has to help with the personal activities and ADLs of ADIs, inclusive of bathing, dressing, grooming, mobility, helping with toilet needs, and incontinence. Toileting is reported to be very stressful for caregivers. Paid care givers have reported how stressful it is to take care of people with dementia in nursing homes. One girl who was a nursing assistant in a nursing home in Phoenix, stated that she was giving up her job since she cannot handle the foul smell of urine and feces. "It is gross, I feel like throwing up; to clean this old lady is difficult because her feces (excrement) is all over the bed and her clothes. I cannot even eat my food thinking of this, I get headache, stomach pain and I feel depressed."

Only a few people can handle this situation but how long? The attrition rate may be very high and this will indirectly affect the patient and different programs that are floated to serve the ADIs. Toilet habits can be physiologically conditioned depending on the physical status of the patient.

Breakfast is an important meal of the day. Get the ADIs participate in the type of meals they like to have. All the meals should be nutritional and palatable. Some of the foods may not agree with the patient and therefore CG may have to consult an expert in the field. If the ADI is living in an Assisted Living facility, the CG in consultation with the ADI may shop for groceries, and prepare meals. When necessary provide transportation. Do not leave the ADI alone anywhere. CG must be present while the ADI is having a meal. Patient can choke on food and may even behave strangely like putting food on their heads or throw food around.

Medication must be administered on schedule and medicines should be locked up.

Mobility needs: ADIs who live in their own homes also will need assistance in moving around, sitting down, getting up, and get in and out of bed. Since ADIs mobility gradually reduces with aging, the CG must be at hand to help the patient.

Patients tend to wander around if they are mobile. They can get out of their homes and hospitals without being noticed. Patient may get out of the bedroom and wander around in the home. ADIs may have visual spatial difficulties and thus may knock around objects in space and get hurt. The patient may enter the kitchen and handle kitchen knife and not knowing what to do with it. Patient may start an oven with the intention to cook but may not carry out the next step in cooking because of cognitive difficulties. Doors will have to be locked lest the patient is out and wander. All the things that are physically not safe will have to be secured. ADI getting lost is a great fear of the family members. Some individuals with AD wander around the premises of the hospitals and someone has to bring the ADI back to her/his room.

The tile makers of India have to keep older people in mind when they manufacture tiles, the texture, color and the size. Non-skidding tiles will have to be installed in the homes since older people are likely to slip and fall down injuring themselves. Developers and promoters of flats for older people will have to design the bedrooms, bathrooms, kitchen and other rooms keeping in mind the safety of the older people.

ADIs need the same protection that a toddler may need. ADIs will need Baby Monitoring System if one can afford it. Other precautions are driveway safety, electrical safety, fire safety where electronic gadgets are installed. Alzheimer's association of USA has recommended the following precautions to protect AD patients. Do not allow the AD patients to venture out on their own. The ADI's sense of direction is very poor. They can easily get lost. Do not leave the AD patient alone when you are out with her/him. Keep very close watch of the patient. Keep the car keys hidden away from the AD patient if the patient is out with you in the car.

The home should be rearranged for the benefit of the AD patients since they are likely to knock against furniture and hurt themselves. They tend to fall down easily and break their brittle bones. Doors must be well secured with the patient in mind.

To take care of an ADI is as difficult as taking care of a toddler. One has to use common sense as to how to protect someone who is not able to assess situations and behave appropriately. Kitchen and bathroom are dangerous places for ADIs. Remove the lock on the bathroom door; install grab bars and rails around the bathtub, toilet and sink. Lower the temperature of the water heater to avoid burns. Remove electrical appliances from the bathroom and away from the water.

ADI must have her/his autonomy as well as safety but do not overdo it since these patients are your loved ones. They have feelings and emotions. ADIs, who are not able to talk, sometimes communicate with tears.

AD patients are at risk for wandering, the ADIs restlessness is a good indicator that they may go astray. They tend to pace, and make repetitive movements. Sense of direction may be poor and thus can get confused even in their own homes to find the bathroom or bedroom. They may be seeking for familiar people. They may not be able to complete work they are attempting to do but may continue repeating the movements. Need instructions written in large letters posted all over the home if the patient has progressed to a moderate to severe level of Alzheimer's. These will contain instructions and directions that will be beneficial for the AD patient. At the Thanksgiving dinner at J's, he brought his father. Senior J was very restless, did not utter a word, socially and emotionally he was distant. He looked lost with a vacant look on his face. Suddenly, he got up and walked fast only to sit in the car. J would bring him back from the car but his father would walk back to the car and sit in the front seat of the car quietly and did not utter a word. This went on for some time till the son took him back to his flat. This was my first encounter with an AD in an informal situation. The restlessness was a message given to his son to take him back to his home.

Since then, I have been meeting Alzheimer's individuals in social situations.

A friend of mine wanted to meet her old friends in San Diego when we were in California to attend a neuropsychological conference. She told me that the man of the house suffers from Alzheimer's. This gentleman was sociable and filled up the gaps of memory of his wife and my friend. He arranged for dinner on a ship. I did not see in him any cognitive disorder or difficulty to communicate. Finally, I asked my friend as to how he got the diagnosis of Alzheimer's! Some of the psychologists who make Alzheimer's diagnosis do not have the educational background and training in clinical psychology/neuropsychology.

In moderately advanced cases, the following may be kept in mind:

1. **Identify causes of problem behavior:** The problem behavior is generally due to strange situations. The ADI may not be able to discuss the situation with caregiver because of communication difficulty.
2. **Create calm and soothing surrounding:** Modify the surroundings to reduce potential stressors. The CG themselves must maintain calmness and be pleasant. Exercise is one of the best stress-relievers. Encourage simple activities that the patient enjoyed in the past. Play soothing music to relax both the patient and the caregiver. Encourage the patient to interact with other people. There are many forms of exercises these days to make ADIs to be active even if the movements are simple.
3. **Disorientation:** It can make a patient wander around. This has to be handled with the consultation of a trained doctor in the field. Australia has special police team to find the missing people.
4. **Manage rummaging and hiding things:** Protect your property and protect the ADI from harming themselves.
5. **Manage belligerence, anger and aggressive behavior:** Do not react to ADIs behaviors. Distract them or

seek help. Communication difficulties will make ADIs manifest distress.

6. **Manage hallucinations and delusions:** Hallucinations may be due to failing senses. The CG has to maintain sameness and calmness for the benefit of the ADI, to help reduce hallucinations and delusions. Violent movies and other situations that are out of character can produce hallucinations and delusions. Caregiver has to be very patient with the ADI and will need reassurances. ADI can get very suspicious and will accuse of people around them of stealing their things. Try to divert their attention from the topic.
7. **Manage sleep problems:** Brain disease often disrupts the sleep-wake cycle. ADIs may be restless, afraid and confused in the night. To maintain calmness in the patient keep regular sleep schedule; keep night light on; increase physical activity during daytime. If the day is enjoyable the ADI probably will have good night sleep.
8. **The eating problem:** Offer food that the patient really likes and can digest; monitor chewing and swallowing since they may choke. One AD patient put the food on her head during lunch; another patient threw the food at another patient. The caregiver's presence is vital during such events.
9. Maintain physical and mental health of the Care givers.

Respite care provides relief to those who care for individuals with Alzheimer's disease or other dementias. Time away from caregiving responsibilities is essential to their own health and allows them to refresh and reduce caregiver stress. An In-Home Respite Volunteer may play a board game or any game with the patient. The patient may be directed to choose the game to make the patient comfortable.

In-Home Social Respite Program

The trained respite volunteers visit the ADIs home to spend time with them for a few hours every other week. Volunteers provide in-home socialization, supervision and meaningful activity for the individual with dementia. This can include reminiscing about the past, listening to music, playing a game, going for a walk, reading aloud, participating in a craft and other activities. The cost for in-home respite in USA is $10 or less per visit and is based on income.

Social Group Respite Programming in USA

The social group respite program allows the person with dementia to exercise their independence and connect with new friends while participating in group activities. This occasion frees the caregiver some free time to meet with friends, go shopping or do things around the house or whatever the CG chooses to do. The social group respite is conducted in a group setting with several respite volunteers and individuals with dementia in a safe location in the community.

What is an Assisted Living Facility?

Assisted living (AL) is a form of long-term care that promotes self-direction and participation in decisions-making. As a model of supportive housing, assisted living emphasizes independence, individuality, privacy, dignity, and choice. It was initially developed to fill the gap between community-based services that support seniors living at home and nursing homes. Assisted living generally places a greater emphasis than nursing homes on preserving "home-like" qualities such as control over one's personal space. Assisted living is growing rapidly, both because it offers an attractive option to seniors seeking assistance while maintaining independence. This is preferable, because of the costs associated with traditional long-term care institutions which are prohibitive for many.

In USA, assisted-living facilities for people with Alzheimer's disease are often referred to as "Special Care Units" or SCUs. SCUs are staffed with individuals who are specially trained to work with people who have Alzheimer's. As such, the environment is designed to be very safe and comfortable, and the activities are designed to benefit the Alzheimer's patients.

SCUs can differ in the level of care they provide along the continuum of the disease. For instance, some assisted living facilities will accept people with Alzheimer's until they need skilled care (nursing home care) whereas others will only accept people who are in the early stages of the disease.

Nursing homes also known as skilled nursing facilities, care for individuals who require 24-hour nursing supervision.

There are two types of care provided in nursing homes in USA. They are:

1. Skilled Care (also known as "sub-acute" or "Medicare occupancy")
2. Long-term Care (also known as "Intermediate Care") as defined by Fisher Centre.

Skilled Care entails services that can be rendered only by a doctor, licensed nurse, physical therapist, occupational therapist, speech and language therapist, social worker or respiratory therapist. It usually follows a hospital visit involving a short-term stay, during which the patient receives nursing care and/or therapy until he or she is stable enough to return home. Due to the skilled nature of the care, it is covered by medicare and secondary insurance for up to 100 days. Beyond that, the services must be paid for privately.

In USA, Long-term Care is appropriate for the individual who can no longer take care of himself or herself and will continue to require a high level of care for the remainder of his or her lifetime. Such care may include help with any "activity of daily living" such as bathing, dressing, transferring (moving from one place to another), toileting, eating and walking. Medicare does not cover this type of care. However, when the individual's financial resources are exhausted, the state-funded source (Medicaid) will supplement the cost. If the nursing home does not accept state funding, one must find another facility that will that accept state funding. Unfortunately, most nursing homes have waiting lists for people entering the facility under state funding. Planning ahead with an appropriate strategy may help the patient and family avoid these conflicts.

Even after moving the patient to Assisted Living Residences or nursing homes, the caregivers continue to help with financial and legal affairs; make arrangement for medical care and provide emotional support. Some caregivers continue to help with bathing, dressing and some ADLs. Caregivers of people with AD provide care for a longer time on average than caregiver of older adults with other conditions.

Hospice

People with AD will have difficulties to meet Hospice eligibility requirements. Hospice is traditionally an option for people whose life expectancy is six months or less, and involves palliative care (pain and symptom relief) rather than ongoing curative measures, enabling one to live last days to the fullest, with purpose, dignity, grace and support. An AD patient may live for many years.

Impact of Caregiving

ADIs symptoms are what the caregivers have to deal with for 24 hours. They have to deal with memory disturbances, orientation, concentration comprehension and communication. As the AD progresses, the person's behavior and personality changes. In some cases, it is very difficult for caregivers to communicate with the patients. The doctor's notes and nurse's notes of nursing homes in USA invariably suggest that the patient is in bed, comprehension is poor, memory is poor, suffers from psychological problems and physical illness. Caregivers and the patient may share emotions, experiences, and memories. This relationship will be an added strain on the CG. A few CGs may continue to lend their services to the ADIs even after the patients are admitted to a nursing home.

The physical and emotional impact of dementia cargiving is estimated to result in 8.7 billion in increased health care costs in the USA. CG can produce metabolic syndrome which will have detrimental effects on health.

There are programs in India to take care of these people and the government spends a meager amount for health care of the dementia patients. Most of the middle class individuals will not be able to meet the expenses. Health cost is very high in USA and I do not have an actual cost incurred by the Government of India to help the AD.

"The national programme (India) for the healthcare of the elderly was being implemented in 100 select districts of 21 states. Besides, eight regional geriatric centres are being funded for the development of dedicated geriatric departments. For this programme, ₹ 150 crore (1.5 billion) will be allotted. The government will also mainstream the department of AYUSH—Ayurveda, Yoga, Unani, Siddha and Homoeopathy—through the national health mission. For this programme ₹ 1,069 crore, will be allotted." Budget 2013-14.

High health cost for instance in California and Florida is as follows:

States	No. of AD and higher health	Hours unpaid	Value of unpaid	Cost of living	Other Dementias
Florida	$ 998684	$1,137,301,634	$13,784,095,810	$ 594,293,482	
California	$1,507,396	$1,716,623,053	$20,805,471,403	$ 785,082,435	

The cost for the following services as of 2011 are as follows:

Per Year	Per day $	Per Year
Home care	168	
Adult Day Centers	70	
Assisted Living care	3477	$41724 per year
Nursing Home: Private room	239	$87235
Semi Private	214	$78,110
AD Charges are Higher	215	$91615
Semi Private for AD	222	$81030

US cost for care of dementias is estimated to be $200 billion in 2012 to 1.1 trillion in 2050. The cost is met by private insurance companies, medicare, medicaid and out of individual's savings. Long-term care insurances pay only 9 per cent. Out of pocket payment is prohibitive. Medicare Part D pays for prescription drugs. Hospice care is estimated to be

$1749 per person. It is projected that the cost will increase to 1.1 trillion by 2050.

The dementia report 2010 a study that was conducted in India by ARDSI offers the following:

In 2009 it was estimated that the societal cost of dementia for India to range between INR 451 to 657 billion as direct cost. The direct cost per person per year is INR 198,197 (USD 4,561.5).

Services for people with dementia inclusive of AD:

The AD and Related Disorders Society in India (ARDSI) was established in 1992. This has 14 chapters in India.

Cost of dementia in India as of 2010 is:

Societal cost	INR	147 billion
Informal care	INR	88.9 billion
Direct individual cost	INR	46.8 billion

The total cost per person with dementia is: INR 43285 ($925)

India is currently spending INR 15 to 16000 crores per year for care of PWD (persons with dementia). The family's cost in care giving is very high. Government has to plan and provide services, infrastructure, building and training at every level. There are several centers in India to serve the AD. These centers are called memory clinics. Most of them are in Kerala.

The ARDSI' Activities and its Services at Kerala State, India:

The Cochin chapter has modeled after USA and UK programs for the Alzheimer's. The drawback for India is the lack of financial resources (personal communication). The programs are run from rented places. The chapter is lacking in funds to run the program. It needs vans to pick up the patients, funds to pay the employees, a building to run conferences, to educate the general population, need educated volunteers, facilities and resources to run various programs to improve cognitive abilities, social interactions and networking.

The memory clinics need innovative programs like exercises/ Yoga for older people, games, entertainments and various therapies including social interactions programs may be helpful for them to be happy for a short while. Laughing therapy is recommended but the ADIs may lack the cognitive abilities to comprehend the context of reference. Children can be very therapeutic and can be facilitators to make Alzheimer's patient's life happier. Pets as an adjunct to therapy will be good for older people but not necessarily for ADIs.

Catholic nuns run homes in Chennai for the poor and sick. Some of them suffer from Alzheimer's. They get very good care. The nuns keep AD patients very clean, and are well fed. The nuns attend to their physical and emotional needs. Even though these patients are terminally ill, the care is such that the patients' feelings and emotions are well protected. These sick patients have feelings and protecting those feelings will contribute to better health. There are only two Belgium nuns at present at this facility and they are old as well. This is more the Mother Teresa model.

Some of the spouses of my colleagues and professors suffer from Alzheimer's. They are physicians, psychiatrists, professors, and psychologists in USA. They are having difficulties to cope with their Alzheimer's spouses. Early distressful emotion they saw in their spouses is change in moods and change in personality. "She is getting angry for no reason, her behavior is unpredictable, keeping vigil on my spouse is telling upon my health. Sometimes I feel like running away." Minneapolis in Minnesota, USA, has facilities where the AD patient can live in one part of the treatment facility and the spouse can live in another part of the building leading normal life. One physician wrote to say that hospitalization is very expensive and is prohibitive to keep his spouse in a nursing home. He said that he is stressed out to a point that he is not able to do his work efficiently as before, and is having difficulty coping with the situation. The ultimate question they have is how to financially cope with taking care of their loved ones. They expect the government to support them with the care of the ADIs. USA has planned well to cater to the needs of ADIs. Developing countries have a long way to go.

Ultimately, it is a societal issue. Despite of all the researches in the area, there is only a dim hope that there will be a medicine that will cure the AD. (Will medicine be a cure?) If there is no medicine in sight, then the neuroscientists will have to look into alternatives like how to prevent AD ever occurring in people. Then the corollary question is "how can old age be prevented?" Some scientists are pursuing this area.

A friend of mine, passed away recently after suffering from Alzheimer's. She belonged to a physician's family. The family gave a glimpse into their trials and tribulations, anxiety, depression, and mental agony. The family is highly educated and educated on this topic. The patient was cared for mainly by Mayo Clinic. The following is quoted from the letter I received from the patient's husband who is a physician. "There are few disorders that can be more devastating for the patient and the caregiver. Over time the involved individual loses all his/her bodily functions. Awareness for the individual is devastating. Since there is no effective management, my family and I suffered immensely. My wife suffered from anxiety, depression, intense fear and pain. My wife's will set out how she wished not to receive Life Saving support including IVs when her physicians determined that no therapeutic measures (known) existed. At the Hospice she finally began to feel at peace. Medications employed were narcotic (Dilaud), Anxiolytic (a benzodiazepine) and finally Phenobarbital. With this medical regimentation, my wife no longer felt the fear, restlessness, and pain (her hospitalization was precipitated by a compound fracture of her right distal tibia, fibula and dislocation of her talus and foot). The latter was dealt with sedation and closed reduction in the Emergency Dept. And her fractures required general anesthetic and an orthopedist to internally fixate the fractures with orthopedic appliances. She was in a cast through the remainder of her life. After three days in the acute hospital setting with family in attendance, she continued with such careful assistance in the acute Health South Rehabilitation Hospital until February the 13th 2014. She was transferred to the Hospice facility on March 5th. She received additional palliative care (no IVs) until she passed away on March 14th at 5:15 AM."

This physician is very concerned about all the patients and patient care. "Adequate caregiver services are essential to help maintain the client's general health. Physical abuse of elderly and Alzheimer's patients by caregivers, nurses, nurse's assistants are worrisome for families of patients. The health system has to improve in patient's care." (*Note*: Physician planned to take a trip with friends to Ireland in September but physician became very depressed, and with sleep apnea. Currently in treatment.)

Herzfeld from USA brought his AD parents to Pondicherry, India, for treatment and care. He rented a home and found staff and helpers to take care of his parents. His father's income was $2000 a month. He found a professional who could give his parents a much higher standard of care than would have been possible in USA with his father's income of $2000 (£1200) a month. In India that paid for their rent, a team of caregivers, a cook, a valet for his father, nurses to be with his mother 12 hours a day, six days a week, a physiotherapist and a masseuse and drugs (costing a fifth of US price), and also allowed them to put some money away. Herzfeld however does not recommend this path to everyone. He believes that India could teach the USA and UK a lot about care of the elderly. "In America, health care is done for profit...." This is Herzfelds experiences.

In the United States, most of the large multi-facility providers are publicly owned and managed as for-profit businesses. There are exceptions; the largest operator in the US is the Evangelical Lutheran Good Samaritan Society, a not-for-profit organization that manages 6531 beds in 22 states, according to a 1995 study by the American Health Care Association. Given the choice, most elders would prefer to continue to live in their own homes (aging in place).[1-2] Unfortunately, majority of elderly people gradually lose functioning ability and require either additional assistance in the home or a move to an elder care facility.[3–4] The adult children of these elders often face a difficult challenge in helping their parents make the right choices. Assisted living is recommended for the elderly who need assistance with everyday tasks, and costs less than home care; however, home care services may allow seniors to live in their own home for a longer period of time.

One relatively new service in the United States that can help keep the elderly in their homes longer is respite care.

Australia

Aged care in Australia is designed to make sure that every Australian can contribute as much as possible toward their cost of care, depending on their individual income and assets. This means that residents pay only what they can afford, and the Commonwealth government pays what a resident cannot.

The review conducted by Australian Statutory Authority concluded that approximately 80 per cent of care for older Australians is informal care provided by family, friends and neighbors. Around a million people received government-subsidized aged care services, most of these receiving low-level community care support, with 160,000 people in permanent residential care. Expenditure on aged care by all governments in 2009-10 was approximately $11 billion.[5, 6]

Due to Australia's aging population, the issue of aged (elderly) care has been highlighted as a key concern for the next 20 years. KPMG.

Medicare Records

In Canada, such privately run for-profit facilities also exist, but they must compete with government-funded public facilities run by each province's or territory's Ministry of Health. In these care homes, elderly Canadians pay for their care on a sliding scale based on annual income. The scale that they are charged on depends on whether they utilize "Long Term Care" or "Assisted Living". For example, commencing in January 2010 seniors living in British Columbia's government subsidized "Long Term Care" (also called "Residential Care") will pay 80 per cent of their after tax income unless their After Tax Income is less than $16,500. The "Assisted Living" tariff is calculated more simply as 70 per cent of the after tax income.

Hospice and Palliative Care

The Essential Guide (2nd ed.), CRC Press.[7] India's cultural view of elderly care is similar to that of most eastern countries.

Parents are typically cared for by their children into old age, most commonly by their sons. It should be noted that in these countries, elderly citizens, especially men, are viewed in very high regard. Traditional values demand honor and respect for older, wiser people. Eightieth birthday of men are celebrated on a large scale in south India. India is facing the same problem as many developing nations in that its elderly population is increasing tremendously, with a current estimate of 90 million over the age of 60. Using data on health and living conditions from the India's 60th National Sample Survey, a study found that almost a quarter of the elderly reported poor health. Reports of poor health were clustered among the poor, single, lower-educated and economically inactive groups.

Article 41 of the Indian Constitution states that elderly citizens will be guaranteed social security support for health care and welfare.[8] A section of the 1973 Criminal Procedure Code, alluding to its traditional background, mandates that children support their parents if they no longer can themselves. NGOs, however, are prevalent in Indian elderly care, providing homes and volunteer care, but governmental policies and organizations are more popular.[9-11]

Medical (Skilled Care) versus Non-medical (Social Care)

Promoting Independence in the Elderly

Promoting independence in self-care can provide older adults with the capability to maintain independence longer and can leave them with a sense of achievement when they complete a task unaided. Those older adults who require assistance with activities of daily living are at a greater risk of losing their independence with self-care tasks as dependent personal behaviors are often met with reinforcement from caregivers. Caregivers must allow older patients to maintain as much independence as possible and function on their own. While they may need supervision, encourage them in their efforts since maintaining independence can provide them with a sense of accomplishment and the ability to maintain independence longer. Feelings of helplessness and futility can cause rebellion due to frustrations. The promotion and maintenance of independence is one of the most important aspects of caring.

Special Care 4 U

"As a Christian run company it practices Christian Principles that is based on the new commandment given by Jesus to love each other." That love is best demonstrated in the ways that it cares and treats each other. The CG is chosen very carefully.

The Special Care 4 U states, "We have staff that are willing to live in your own home providing you with full time help and support that might prevent you from going into residential care or nursing homes. All of our staff have lots of experience for helping people to live in their own homes and have very loving and caring. Our live in staff can be everything you need from cleaning, cooking, shopping, ironing, helping you bath and dress yourself, taking medicines or taking you out to different places."

ARDSI (Alzheimer's and Related Disorders Society of India) is one of the main resources for dementia caregivers in India.

ARDSI's activities are devoted exclusively to help dementia patients and their families. They are involved in dementia and caregiving awareness activities. They are involved with developing services, training family members and professionals, and undertaking research. They run several help lines to provide information on Alzheimer's and caregiving.

Swapna Kishore was a caregiver and now a blogger and a resource person. Her blogs contain the following information:

"These homes have strict rules/conditions. There are many old age homes/respite care/assisted living/ashrams for elders as such. The following are her comments on facilities that take care of dementia patients:

Most refuse admission outright. Many non-specialized old age homes tell families to take back the patient if the patient shows agitation or strange behaviours or gets bedridden. For example, night pacing or agitation can earn expulsion very fast.

Even old age homes that accept dementia patients often have no staff training for handling such patients. Most old age homes are not designed for patients who can harm themselves. Patient accidents and injuries are therefore high.

While some families report good experiences especially if the facility is designed for dementia patients and staffed with trained, sensitive people, other families are not always happy. Here are some problems mentioned to me by families, volunteers, and even ex-staff of such home—(I'm excluding normal problems any old age home may have like poor hygiene, bad food, and rooms left dirty, rude staff, and so on). She added:

- Patients being tied up by staff so that the staff can sleep/go for movies.
- Patients falling off beds at night because the night-duty staff stayed awake during the day and was dozing and the patients wanted to go to the bathroom.
- Patients get yelled at by frustrated attendants, and are called all sorts of names and accused of misbehaviour.
- Rough handling, visible bruises on the arm and so on.
- Patients are mixed with normal elders, frustrating for both parties, and the patients end up yelling at/getting yelled at by these normal elders because the patients behaved in odd ways and the normal elder does not understand it is dementia.
- Patients are moved between rooms without families being told, something very disorienting for the patient.
- Frequent staff changes and not passing on patient case history across staff members.
- Frequent summoning of family members to "explain" to the patient not to "misbehave".

- Being asked to take back patient, often at short notice. (The above features are reported in US as well but not to this extent)."

All the above-mentioned features are reported in other developed countries as well and not specific to India.

So finding a good old age home that accepts and cares well for dementia patients is tough. Finding a home that will continue to care for the patient as the patient deteriorates and gets more disoriented and dependent and bedridden is very tough. Being at peace with the decision, doing a smooth transition, and remaining free from worry is yet another challenge. Some people do strike it lucky and find a good place for their loved one. I have no overall numbers for India. This is, frankly, an unorganized and unregulated service as of now. It is a patchy service in supply and quality, with individuals and agencies involved, and some good but many horror stories attached.

Family Support

Researchers from the Oxford Institute of Aging have produced a leaflet full of ideas on how to maintain relationships across the generations when a grandparent has dementia. Although dementia affects everyone in a family, most research focuses on the person with dementia or their main carer. In the Oxford study, parents, grandparents and children from six families were all interviewed, as were some of the professionals involved in supporting them. Based on the interviews, the researchers found the following:

Strong Identity

Most of the grandparents with dementia who took part in the research had a strong sense of their identity as a grandparent, with their role remaining important to them. Grandparents in India have very special importance and position in the family. Even when dementia had affected verbal skills, grandparents were still able to express their identity through interactions at an emotional level such as showing happiness to see their grandchildren and at being able to share activities.

The Child's View

Maintaining the relationship:

To ensure that children continue to spend time and engage with their grandparents, researchers recommend that adults provide practical support to help them. One of the suggestions is to discuss in advance what they might talk about during the visit such as a recent experience.

Grandparents might also need suggestions or encouragement about what activities they can participate in with their grandchild. (Teenagers who volunteer to work in mental hospitals, during summer vacation relate well with the patients and vice versa.)

Professor Harper is convinced that for many children, particularly those who are a bit older, being responsible in some minor way for the care and support of a grandparent with dementia can bring a tremendous sense of worth and responsibility.

Due to Australia's ageing population, the issue of aged (elderly) care has been highlighted as a key concern for the next 20 years.

Wikipedia the free encyclopedia and ARDSI (Alzheimer's and Related Disorders Society of India) maybe referred for more information on this topic.

NOTES

1. Department of Health and Aging-Aged Care Australia. Retrieved 2010-11-22.
2. Elderly care or elder care is directed to the fulfillment of the special needs and requirements that are unique to senior citizens. This broad term encompasses such services as assisted living, adult day care, long term care, nursing homes (often referred to as residential care), hospice care, and home care. Because of the wide variety of elderly care found nationally, as well as differentiating

cultural perspectives on elderly citizens, cannot to be limited to any one practice.

3. Gross, Jane (July 2008) coined the phrase "Aging in Place" which meant that many retiree and pre-retirees have their hearts set on ageing in their own current homes as long as possible before having to move to a secure facility for older people who needs supervision and care.
4. Gericare Finder, "Senior Care" or Geriatric care management (also known as "Aging Life Care™", "elder care management", "senior health care management" and "professional care management") is the process of planning and coordinating care of the elderly and others with physical and/or mental impairments to meet their long term care needs, improve their quality of life, and maintain their independence for as long as possible. It entails working with persons of old age and their families in managing, rendering and referring various types of health and social care services. Geriatric care managers accomplish this by combining a working knowledge of health and psychology, human development, family dynamics, public and private resources and funding sources, while advocating for their clients throughout the continuum of care. For example, they may assist families of older adults and others with chronic needs such as those suffering from Alzheimer's disease or other dementia.

   (Geriatric care management https://en.wikipedia.org/wiki/Geriatric_care_management)
5. *New York Times* (2008) subsequently interviewed Jane Gross and wrote an article on her theme "Aging in Place" called "Faced with Caring" (2008). Hence the term "Aging in Place" became popular. The next stage in caring of older people is known as Assisted Living.
6. Productivity Commission (2011). Caring for older Australians. Overview. Canberra: Productivity Commission.
7. Stephen, Connor (2009). Hospice and Palliative Care: The Essential Guide (2nd ed.) CRS. p. 202.
8. India: Care and Support for the Elderly in India.

9. Help Age. "http//www.helpageindia.org/about-us.plp" India 2009.
10. http//www.futurehealthsystem.org/publications/hetergeneity-in-self-assessed-health-statu-among-t-the-elder.htm
11. "The Elderly in India", *Asia-Pacific Journal of Public Health*.

REFERENCES

Connor, Stephen (2009). *Hospice and Palliative Care: The essential Guide* (2nd ed.) CRS. p. 202.

Department of Health and Aging Aged Care Australia. Retrieved 2010-11-22.

Elderly in India: *Asia-Pacific Journal of Public Health*.

Faced with Caregiving: *New York Times*. Retrieved 2008-07-26.

Gericare Finder. "SeniorCare". Retrieved September 2012. http//en.wikipedia.org/wiki/

Gross, Jane (July 2008) What is aging in Place? AgeInPlace.com

Help Age "http//www.helpageindia.org/about-us.plp" India 2009.

http//www.futurehealthsystem.org/publications/hetergeneity-in-self-assessed-health-statu-among-t-the-elder.htm

India: Care and Support for the Elderly in India.

MedLine Plus. Retrieved 26 September 2012: Assisted Living.

(2011). Caring for older Australians. Overview. Canberra: Productivity Commission.

9

Prevention

Alzheimer's has no cure so far but cure may not loom large at a distance since neuroscientists are conducting research from every possible angle including cure with stem cells.

Preventive measures to ward off Alzheimer's: Most of the researchers suggest lifestyle choices to protect the health of the brain.

Regular Exercise

It is fashionable for people to go to spas these days. However, Nature offers abundance of facilities for exercise. Walk, jog in a park, listening to birds, watching flowers and trees, listening to the rustle of the leaves of eucalyptus trees, greeting healthy people on the way. People who grow up in mountainous areas spent time exploring the hills, the trees, the shrubs, rare fruit trees, flowering plants, the nests of birds and bird watching and exploring beautiful things in nature. All the five senses are also stimulated. Regular exercise is very beneficial to maintain normal health. Take a walk along the beach and listen to the changing sounds of the tides and how they change their moods.

Alzheimer's may be encouraged to exercise since it relaxes, induces happy mood, and above all improves cognitive abilities. Yoga classes are streamlined for older people in India. The participants socialize after the classes and often are in touch with new friends on the phone or they get together for a cup of coffee. They plan events to attend like carnatic music, theatre productions and other social activities.

Mediterranean diet is highly recommended for westerners but for most of the Indians, vegetarian food with variety of pulses, grains, vegetables and spices are not only palatable but they consider them to be very nutritious and healthy. Omega 3 is available in many foods including Flax seed and variety of other seeds like sesame.

Eat heart healthy diet: Berries and green leafy vegetables should be part of every one's diet for brain-protective regimen. Indian foods in general include variety of whole grains, pulses and variety of vegetables including leafy ones, gourds, rhizomes, fruits of the season, nuts and seeds. The Indian sweets are made out of milk products and they come in different tastes and shapes.

"A healthy meal is one that includes all the six tastes, qualitatively and quantitatively in the order of sweet (mudra) as in rice, ghee; sour (amla) as in citrus fruits; salty (lavana); pungent or hot (katur) as in chilly, spices; pitta (bitter) as in bitter gourd, spinach; astringent (kashaya) as in buttermilk, tea. Do not end with a dessert. Every day, make sure you eat a vegetable or fruit of the three colors—orange, red and green including watery vegetables." This is the advice of Dr. Seshadri, veteran ayurvedic consultant, and professor. Majority of Indians are vegetarians and the variety of foods is beyond imagination.

Enjoy daily cups of tea. Regular consumption of green tea may enhance memory and mental alertness and slow brain aging. Black tea is more widely consumed than green tea worldwide. India is the largest producer of black tea. Polyphenolic compounds present in black tea can protect cells and tissues from oxidative stress by scavenging free radicals. Theanine present in black tea increases alpha brain wave activity resulting in calmer state of mind and it reduces stress. Being a very high source of antioxidants, black tea is said to slow down aging process and age induced diseases. Research suggests coffee and caffeine help suppress the increase in amyloid plaques in the brain and inflammation (Tea Board 2013-14).

Folic acid, vitamin B12, vitamin D, magnesium, and fish oil are believed to preserve and improve brain health. Researchers at Oxford University found that lack of B12 actually shrinks the brain and a shortage can lead to brain atrophy by ripping away, myelin, a fatty protective sheath around neurons. It can also trigger inflammation, another destroyer of brain cells. One may need 500 to 1000 mcg of vitamin B12 daily after the age of 40.

Maintain Cognitive Abilities

Learn something new every day if possible to keep the brain active. In US the adult education programme keep older people engaged in some activity they are interested in. Painting, chess, bridge, computers, making jewellery and so on are some of the activities that are good for cognitive reserve.

Memory

All the features of memory have to be trained on a regular basis. Recite favourite poems; relearn Shakespeare or Wordsworth or Keats or whoever your favourite poets are. Go back to KG and remember what you learnt. Learn the flags of the different countries; learn the names of the different states in India and languages of each state. One can make a game out of it. If the state is mentioned, associate it with the language of the state or their attire. There are very interesting memory games on the Internet to play tapping different aspects of the brain. The game becomes very entertaining if an adult plays in the company of a child 6-7 years of age. The newspapers *Hindu* and *The Times of India* in Chennai put out pencil-paper games every day in the form of puzzles, games, riddles, general knowledge and so on. Do crossword puzzles, scrabble, play Chinese checkers and any such games that you like. Child's playful behaviours will be an added incentive to remember the strategies. Work on a project of your choice. This is helpful for abstract intelligence and memory. Explore something new to create new brain pathways. Internet offers entertainment of an intellectual nature. Watch geographic magazine, Discovery channel, cooking channels. Food and cooking fascinate many people. Interest in cooking keeps many active and happy. Food and socialization are intertwined.

Sleep

Sleep is very important for normal functioning. Lack of sleep is toxic to brain cells. Bed time has to be scheduled and the conditions for sleep must be conducive for a good night sleep. Soft soothing music, favourite prayer, someone to say good night are pacifying and comforting before going to sleep. Sleep has surprising powers to protect your brain against memory loss and Alzheimer's. In the private boarding school as the children got ready to go to sleep in the night, Miss Brooks a teacher from England invariably came in to say good night. She would say in a sweet voice "An angel at your head, an angel at your feet, one on the left, one on the right and one above. Good Night children." Children went to sleep calmly. Even now I can hear her say that.

Restorative deep breathing and Yoga poses impact oxygen levels in the brain. Pleasant thoughts, relaxed social and emotional interactions, positive attitudes and stress relieving exercises are vital to maintain overall health; for neurogenesis.

Stress management: Persistent stress reactions triggered by everyday events like work frustration, traffic jams and financial worries can be dangerous. Yoga, Sauna, massage and medicated oil baths keep one rejuvenated. Ayurvedic centers are a big business in India especially in the south, the birthplace of Ayurvedic medicine. Walking and jogging in the parks are beneficial in the sense that and one can have free oxygen as well.

Attend clubs if they are available for socialization and participation in various activities. In India, the clubs are established for the benefits of rich and famous to promote their business and business contacts. Women from these affluent families get together for lunch mostly. Socialization is rejuvenating and maintains "cognitive reserve". Intermingling with people, sharing ideas, laughing together are good for the brain activity. Avoid anxiety evoking social situations.

Meditation and prayer offer a state of internal peace and serenity. It is peaceful to watch people in prayer in the temples, churches and mosques in India. "The sound of a single church bell is solemn and sublime, while the pealing of several bells more or less in concert is even more majestic sounding. The mighty peal of bells has an effect on our inner sensibilities, awakening our souls from spiritual sleep. "Ringing of bells has spiritual value irrespective of religions. In olden days, people believed that bells, chimes, jingles, cymbals and gongs are commonly said to be good luck and are often used to ward off evil spirits. Could the ringing of bells really exercise spiritual power, enabling some supernatural influence in the natural realm? While some believe and others doubt, there is a reality beyond superstition."

"Cheerfulness keeps up a kind of daylight in the mind, and fills it with a steady and perpetual serenity" (Joseph Addison, 1672-1719).

Some activities that may reduce the risk of developing dementia include:

- Be cheerful and happy to relax your mind.
- Mental stimulation.
- Reading.
- Writing for pleasure.
- Learn another language to speak. There are 20 major languages in India.
- Play musical instruments.
- Take part in adult education courses. Women in India are interested in sewing, knitting, embroidery, quilting, glass painting, jewelry making, pottery and so on.
- Practice memorization.
- Participate in interactive activities swimming.
- Group activities, club activities, plan short trips to exciting places.
- Engage in traditional folk dances, songs and engage in reviving traditional art forms.
- Get involved with cognitive stimulation in order to improve memory, concentration, flexibility of thinking, abilities to solve problem and improve language ability.

- Discuss issues of importance to you with friends, family, and any one knowledgeable about the topic. Get together for a cup of coffee.
- Stimulate the five senses.
- Take part in plays, write your own skits.
- Practice loud laughter away from people lest someone thinks you are mentally deranged.
- Add variety to your routine. Try something new.
- Drop unnecessary commitments. Focus on what matters.
- Avoid situations that drain your energy above all avoid difficult people who make your life miserable.

"There is no evidence that playing 'brain training' computer games reduces the risk of dementia." However, it is fun to engage in such activities. You can read more information about ongoing dementia research on the Alzheimer's Research UK website.

Activities that require one to use all the senses break routines and engage in novel experiences which can create BDNFs (neurotrophins) as explained in the book *Keep Your Brain Alive,* Workman Publishing. BDNF (Brain-derived neurotrophic factor) is a secreted protein that in humans, is encoded by the BDNF gene. It is related to "Nerve growth factor" NGF.

Activities that involve planning ahead like chess, stimulate the frontal lobe activities cricket and basketball train short range spatial skills, used when one walks through a short limited space, like the interior of a house. Activities that combine intellectual and physical demands improve spatial and reasoning skills. Activities like learning a new language or painting require the coordination of multiple regions of the brain.

Physical exercise promotes BDNF (Brain-derived neurotrophic factor).

Games to Train the Brain: A few computer games are free of charge.

Lifestyle strategies that promote neurogenesis and regrowth of brain cells include the following. These entire strategies target a specific gene pathway called BDNF or brain-derived neurotrophic factor, which promotes brain cell growth and connectivity as demonstrated on MRI scans.

Exercise: In a year-long study, individuals who engaged in exercise were actually growing and expanding the brain's memory center one to two per cent per year, whereas typically that center would have continued to decline in volume.

Reducing overall calorie consumption.

Reducing carbohydrate consumption.

Increasing healthy fat consumption.

Increasing your omega-3 fat intake and reducing consumption of damaged omega-6 fats.

Same factors that increase the risk of heart disease can also increase the risk of Alzheimer's disease and vascular dementia. Important factors that may be involved include high blood pressure, high blood cholesterol, excess weight and diabetes. Therefore, it is prudent on the part of everyone to be involved with physical activities, cognitive stimulation, social engagement and sensible diet.

"Dr. Perlmutter, prefers krill oil to omega-3 and 6, since it contains astaxanthin. It belongs to the class of carotenoids, and is very 'focused' on reducing free radical-mediated damage to fat, and the brain is 60 or 70 per cent fat". He also recommends fasting (Dr. Perlmutter, Wikipedia).

Anti-inflammation food: Dark Chocolate: The flavonoids in coco increases blood flow to the brain.

Red wine and green tea contain catechins and clams contain B12. Clams have 98.9 mcg of vitamin B12 in just 100 g serving. Asparagus is high in folate. Many vegetables contain folate. Salmon contains omega-3, Vitamin D and B12; Walnut improves motor and cognitive skills; red cherries have anti-inflammatory properties. Almost all berries reduce brain inflammation. Turmeric is anti-inflammatory and removes plaques from the brain. Quercetin is found in abundance in the skins of apples which protects the brain from damages associated with Alzheimer's disease and other neurodegenerative disorders. Cornell University research found this to be true. Experts from the University of California, San Francisco, said that over 50 per cent of all Alzheimer's cases may be prevented through lifestyle changes. This involves reducing important risk factors, including:

- not smoking
- being physically and mentally active
- combating low education
- properly treating or preventing chronic diseases and conditions such as hypertension (high blood pressure), high blood cholesterol, diabetes, obesity in midlife, and depression.

Many experts believe that controlling cardiovascular risk factors may be the most cost-effective and helpful approach to protecting brain health. Physical exercise, diet, social engagement and intellectual activities contribute to brain health. Suggested Therapies to Prevent Alzheimer's (refer to Chapter 7 on Treatment).

Nature is therapeutic for ADIs. Nature has myriad facets. It changes from minute to minute in front of our eyes. The sea changes its color with the change of weather and depending on the positions of the moon and the sun. Watching sunrise, sunset, full moon and natural phenomena transport people to a state of tranquillity and ecstasy. Watching and being with the birds and butterflies that we share our garden space which afford us with experience of greater feelings of relaxation and a sense of appreciation for the diversity of nature.

Visual Stimulation

Visual stimulation is a good exercise for Alzheimer's patients as well.

As normal individuals, visual stimulation can involve light, color, shape, motion, or a combination of all these features.

A reflection of the sunset and moon on the sea may trigger a memory of a similar sunset in the past. It also stimulates the brain. Enjoy the glorious sunset and the full moon that create a series of changing colors on the mountain. A classic painting may be remembered from a visit to a museum or an art appreciation class in college. A good alternative to feature movies is nature documentaries. The Aurora Borealis with its splendor of colors on display and the frozen Niagara Falls are phenomena of natural beauty to behold. Nature and its vicissitudes help in the treatment and prevention of Alzheimer's.

> "When I admire the wonders of a sunset or the beauty of the moon,
>
> My soul expands in the worship of the creator."
>
> —*Mahatma Ghandi*

Auditory Stimulation

People with Alzheimer's disease may have normal hearing, but they may lose their ability to interpret what they hear accurately. This loss may result in confusion or overstimulation.

Sounds and Music: Nature provides many sounds that are musical to the ear stimulating to the brain. Let the ADIs get out and listen to the sounds of nature. The singing of the birds, the rustle of the leaves, the sound of wind or torrential rain can bring memories of past experiences. This is used in reminiscence therapy. Music is used to grow plants faster and healthier. Music is good for self-enhancement, relaxation and cognition. Farmers play music to their cows and the cows produce more milk. Music makes plants grow faster and healthier. Music is good for all living things including people. Music is soothing and transports individuals to a state of peace and happiness within. Music of one's choice is beneficial to patients who are agitated. The sound of waterfalls and the rustic beauty of the same with water spraying around cooling the rocks and plants are peaceful and exuberant. Natural sounds are probably the best for mood and meditation. A gentle rain, or the wind blowing through magnolia trees, can work wonders for everyone's moods. To stimulate cognition, Western classical or Indian classical music is ideal.

Familiar music is stimulating on several levels, and is a strong and important component of a comprehensive reminiscence therapy. If the patient plays a musical instrument encourage the person to play for the enjoyment of self and others. Sing-Along is fun and can stimulate memory. Many people who have Alzheimer's disease will remember songs, lyrics and enjoy singing them long after other communication skills and memories are gone.

Background Sounds and White Noise

Stimulating sound or music playing in the background while other activities are going on improves the mood, and even the memory of people with all forms of dementia. This background sound can be reminiscence.

Exercise to Music. Physical exercise and reminiscence are two powerful tools for the management of Alzheimer's, and combining the two will undoubtedly result in an enjoyable activity. This is a preventive measure to Alzheimer's. It is very good for the health of normal people as well. India has a large repertoire of folk dances and folk art extending from north to south and east to west. The dances come alive during religious festivities.

Smell

Ambient odors influence and uplift moods, work performance, and many other forms of behavior. This is because of their learned associations and their emotional associations. Find out whether any mood change has occurred, and if so, does this mood change makes one want to do anything in particular.

Study of smell on Alzheimer's: Cardiff University, Professor Tim Jacob, school of Biosciences is studying the olfactory function in humans. "How and why do we smell?" The olfactory bulb is one of the structures of the limbic system and a very ancient part of the brain. The information captured by the sense of smell goes from the olfactory bulb to other structures of the limbic system. The limbic system is also concerned with translating sensory data from the neo-cortex (the thinking brain) into motivational forces for behavior. In any case good smell is relaxing and bad smell is revolting to the senses.

Robert S. Wilson et al. studied olfactory identification and incidence of Mild Cognitive Impairment in old age. They used tests for memory, remembering, ideas, words, symbols and perceptual speed. The researchers concluded that: "Among older persons without manifest cognitive impairment, difficulty in identifying odors predicts subsequent development of MCI."

A poor sense of smell may be one of the earliest signs of Alzheimer's. Now, researchers have shown that the offending culprit may be beta-amyloid, a protein that builds up in a toxic form in the brains of those with the disease. "Cognitive Facilitation Following Intentional Odor Exposure" (Andrew, J. Johnson, 2011).

This paper reviews evidence that, in addition to incidental olfactory pollutants, intentional odor delivery can impact cognitive operations both positively and negatively. Evidence for cognitive facilitation/interference is reviewed alongside four potential explanations for odor-induced effects. It is concluded that the pharmacological properties of odors can induce changes in cognition.

Taste

The patient and/or caregiver should compile a list of foods and spices that have always been enjoyed by the individual. Choose and prepare foods that have an aesthetic appearance and texture. Encourage ADIs to watch cooking shows which might improve their appetite and memories of their favorite dishes.

A chef said: "When I get an idea for a dish, firstly I start to think about flavour combination, then how it's cooked, then what do I serve it on." He further added that some chefs prefer to serve food on white plate. The debate rages on among chefs as to the shape and color of the plates. It is preferable to serve on white so that food is conspicuous. The colour white has implicit associations with feelings of purity, brightness or possibly cleanliness (among many other things I suspect).

The senses of taste and smell are very closely related. If an individual loses some or all of sense of taste, there are things that can be done to make food taste better. Foods can be prepared with a variety of colors and textures. Aromatic herbs and hot spices add more flavour but adding more sugar or salt to foods may be avoided.

ADIs sense of smell and taste can diminish over time. Thus, they may be inclined to eat less or may even refuse to eat.

Taste helps all individuals to recognize when food is good or bad. When an elderly person loses taste, it can cause loss of appetite, weight loss, poor nutrition, weakened immunity, and even death. Use white dishes to help ADI to distinguish the food from the plate. Similarly, use placemats of a contrasting color to help distinguish the plate from the table. Stick with solid colors. Patterned plates, bowls and linens might be confusing.

The theory behind the deterioration of these senses in the elderly person has been covered by scientists but effects on the person's lifestyle along with the dangers associated with such disorders have to be explored. "Flavor enhancement for the elderly and sick can improve food palatability and acceptance, increase lymphocyte counts, reverse or slow functional decline, and improve overall quality of life. It also has the potential to compensate for anorexia" (*Postgraduate Medical Journal*, 2005). An additional study found that flavor enhancement for elderly retirement home residents resulted in improved immune status as determined by T and B cell levels and improved grip strength. Taste and odor stimulation has also been shown to increase the rate of salivary IgA in the elderly person (*Postgraduate Medical Journal*, 2006). The findings accord with a burgeoning body of scientific research demonstrating that the human senses interact and combine to form an overall impression of experiences. Taste is no exception. So the sounds we hear, and the shapes and colors we observe, markedly influence the flavor of food and drink.

"It is an area of research only flourishing in recent times," says Dr Costa. "Research", he adds, "is now beginning to explore the influence of cutlery texture on flavour—such as whether a fork or spoon is made of plastic or metal."

"This simple experiment clearly shows that our oral sensors are influenced by what effects of ageing on smell and taste" (J.M. Boyce and G.R. Shone).

Food, Eating and Alzheimer's recommended by Alzheimer's Society: As a person's cognitive functions decline, he or she may become overwhelmed with too many food choices. Patient may forget to eat or may have difficulty with eating utensils.

Nutrition Tips: Provide a balanced diet with a variety of foods; limit foods with high saturated fat and cholesterol. Cut down on refined sugars. Limit foods with high sodium and use less salt.

Possible Causes are Poor Appetite: Not recognizing food; poor fitting dentures; decreased sense of smell and taste; medications; lack of exercise.

Make Meal Times Easier: Limit distractions. Keep the table setting simple. Distinguish food from the plate. Check the food temperature; serve only one or two foods at a time. Be flexible to food preferences.

Give the person plenty of time to eat. Eat together. Keep in mind the person may not remember when or if he or she ate.

Touch

Touch and contact are primary language of compassion, and a primary means for spreading compassion. Alzheimer's disease may lead to decreased sensitivity to touch in some people. This can include a diminished ability to interpret feelings of heat, cold, or pain. Touch is truly fundamental to human communication, bonding, and health. Extensive research by the University of Miami's Touch Research Institute has revealed that human touch has wide-ranging physical and emotional benefits for people of all age groups. Massage is very important to older people for blood circulation and rejuvenation and the feeling of compassion. Touch itself is therapeutic.

Part of what's so amazing about touch is that people can feel all the different textures and temperatures. People can experience different sensations through touching and feeling the soft petals of flowers, soft silk, the bark of a tree, digging the feet into sand on the beach and many such activities. Try not to let a day go by without experiencing pleasant and soothing touch. A consoling touch when one is going through a traumatic experience can be not only consoling but can be healing. Some people practice the healing touch. If the ADI is not able to go out to enjoy, then virtual environments can be created. Computer engineers are working on it.

Fun, Laughter and Games of Ancient Times

Very old indoor games in Tamil Nadu (Chennai) India: *Aadu puli attam* (goat and tiger dance). It is a village game (like chess). Chess also originated in India.

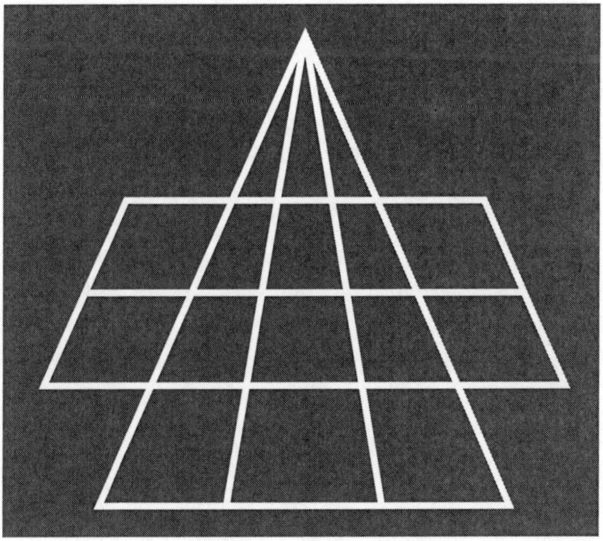

This pattern is drawn on the floor

Poo Parikka Varugirom

Poo parikka varugirom (coming to pluck flowers) is an interesting traditional game played in villages by singing a song which is in question and answer form. This game develops physique, singing, knowing flowers, counting, questioning and answering skill.

Some of the other traditional games are: Pallanguli is played in the southern India. It is called the gambling game by men.

Pachisi: It is a board game that originated in ancient India.

Kankad: This game more popular among girls is played with 5 or 7 stones. Requiring permutations and combinations to increase the difficulty levels. For example, picking one stone from ground while three are in the air and have to catch all of them.

Char Bhar: Mind Boggling game which requires abstract thinking.

Each state in India has its own games and they are usually social group games.

Traditional games act as learning aids. They teach many things. They teach people to accept the process behind 'win and lose', develop sensory skills, count, add, improve motor skills, identify colour, improve hand-eye co-ordination and finally to have fun, naturally people play or watch a game to have fun.

REFERENCES

Andrew, J. Johnson 2011: Cognitive Facilitation Following Intentional Odor Exposure. Memory, remembering ideas, words and symbols and perceptual speed.

Bobson, Roger. Saga. www.saga.co.uk: How smell affects your body and mind.

The HINDU, Chennai. Monday, January 13, 2014. Eat heart healthy diet. *Post Graduate Medical Journal* 2005: Flavor enhancement for the elderly and sick increase lymphocyte counts, reverse or slow functional decline. *Post Graduate Medical Journal* 2006: Flavor enhancement for elderly retirement home residents resulted in improved immune status as determined by T and B cell levels and improved grip strength. Taste and odor stimulation has also been shown to increase the rate of salivary IgA in the elderly person.

Jacob, Tim Prof. School of Biosciences, Cardiff University: The Psychophysiology of smell.

Johnson, Andrew Sensors (Basel) V.11(5)(2011). Cognitive Facilitation Following Intentional Odor Exposure. Memory, remembering ideas, words and symbols and perceptual speed.

Perlmutter, Dr. from Wikipedia: prefers Krill oil to Omega 3 and 6. The consciouslife.com/brain-foods-prevent-dementia-Alzheimer: 9 brain foods that prevent Dementia and Alzheimer's. J.M. Boyce and G.R. Shone: oral sensors are influenced by what effects (texture and color of plates and placemats) of ageing on smell and taste.

Rush University Medical Center Tuesday 23 July, 2013: Eating certain foods may help prevent Alzheimer's disease. "How to prevent Alzheimer's disease and dementia"

University of Miami's Touch Research Institute: Effects of touch therapy (current study), has wide-ranging physical and emotional benefits for people of all age groups.

Wilson Robert, S. et al. (2007): *Arch Gen Psychiatry*. "Olfactory, Identification and Incidence of Mild Cognitive Impairment in Old Age." *Arch Gen Psychiatry*. (2007); 64:802-08.

10

Cognitive Stimulation Therapy/ Habilitation for Mild to Moderate Alzheimer's

Non-pharmacological interventions, and particularly cognition-based interventions, are increasingly being recognized as an important adjunct and, in some cases, alternative to pharmacological treatments for individuals with dementia and those at risk of dementia.

Memory loss is one of the first or more-recognizable signs of dementia. Other early signs may include:

- Repeating questions and repeating on a subject like have you had your water?
- Forgetting words that are very common only if this is frequent. (At times every one forgets words but remember later on.)
- Substituting a word for the intended one for example car for Bar. (Under stress people can interchange words)
- Taking excessive time to complete tasks and probably not completing tasks.
- Misplacing things like car keys or keys to the cupboards frequently and not able to recollect.
- Getting lost even in familiar surroundings, losing directions.

- Unpredictable moods and misinterpreting situations.
- Difficulties to follow directions more often than not and tend to ask what did you say?
- Standing still having forgotten the intended activity.
- Wanting to ask for help but taking a long time to ask for it. (Alzheimer's Society)

Almost all activities of ADI are slowed down and as such do not hasten the person to respond immediately.

Areas to work on are the following:

- Attention, concentration
- Memory
- Language and communication
- Perceptual functions including visual, auditory, olfactory, and gustatory modalities as well as somatosensory systems
- Concept formation and problem-solving
- Planning and organization
- Speed of processing
- Behavior, emotions and personality.

Cognitive Training involves repeated practice on specific tasks which is supposed to improve cognitive processes such as memory and concentration. Cognitive training is the restoration of cognitive deficits. Hand in hand reality orientation has to be instituted with information about time, place or person in order to ease the understanding of the person about surroundings and one's place in them. Both have shown some efficacy improving cognitive capacities. Stimulate activities that are familiar and of interest to the ADIs.

Cognitive Rehabilitation is an individualized approach that builds on strengths and compensates for areas of weakness in order to enhance an individual's ability to participate more fully in everyday activities.

Habilitation and *Rehabilitation* both focus on the act of learning skills. The primary difference between the two is that habilitation focuses on learning new skills on the basis of cognitive reserve whereas rehabilitation focuses on regaining skills that are lost. Both modalities accentuate improvement of performance in everyday life by improving cognitive abilities. There is evidence to support an association between lifelong cognitive stimulation and increased cognitive reserve that may reduce the likelihood of functional cognitive impairments in advanced age [Wilson, Barnes, and Bennett (2003); Wilson et al. (2002); Wilson, R., Barnes, L., and Bennett, D. (2003), Wilson, R.S., Mendes De Leon, C.F., Barnes, L.L., Schneider, J.A. Biennia's, J.L., Evans, D.A., and Bennett, D.A. (2002); K., Barnes, D., Nevitt, M., Lui, L.Y., and Covinsky, K. (2001); Alzheimer's Society].

Cognitive Stimulation is an activity-based therapy that draws upon effective elements of a number of therapies including reality orientation and reminiscence therapy, art, music exercise, pet therapies and any kind of recreational activities. Cognitive stimulation therapy (CST) benefits cognition and quality of life for individuals with dementia. Intervention is provided in a group setting, with focus on global cognitive stimulation, social interaction and implicit learning. Importantly, cognitive stimulation is the only non-pharmacological approach with sufficient evidence to warrant recommendation by the National Institute for Health and Clinical, Excellence (NICE) UK. Research evidence suggests that CST can benefit cognitive function, quality of life, well-being, communication and social interaction. CST has also been recommended by the NICE SCIE Guidelines (2006) for all individuals with mild-moderate dementia. You can read more about CST at www.cstdementia.com

Activities that provide cognitive stimulation ideally target both cognitive and social functioning. Cognitive stimulation can be administered either in a group setting, or can be provided individually by a professional or a family member who is responsible for the AD. It must address individual's specific interests and abilities.

The following are the modifiable lifestyle factors that may potentially enhance cognitive abilities:

- *Thinking*—puzzles, games, reading, writing.
- *Physical*—walk, jog, take arm and leg exercises, move your body by dancing/folk dances.
- *Creative*—arts and crafts, painting, playing music or singing.
- *Social*—socially engaging with family and friends, with people at religious centers, other activity centers.
- *Chores*—everyday routine activities, folding the laundry, setting the table, feeding cats, dogs, birds, and the pets.
- *Daily living*—taking a shower, brushing teeth, eating, getting dressed.

Cognitive stimulation activities include discussion of past and present events and topics of interest. Word games, puzzles, music, and practical activities such as baking or indoor gardening.

Research conducted by NICE suggests that participants who received cognitive stimulation also reported improved quality of life and that they were able to communicate and interact better than before.

Along with reducing the risk of dementia, research suggests that playing mind games can help promote brain health and strengthen critical thinking.

Scrabble requires semantic and short-term memory skills. It mostly uses left brain.

Chess is a left-brain activity. Chess requires skill, intelligence, and planning ability. Chess and mathematics are highly correlated and sharpen memory.

Backgammon is cognitively stimulating. It trains concentration and strategic thinking.

Parcheesi needs the help of both left and right brain hemispheres. It improves eye-hand coordination.

Chinese checkers uses both brain hemispheres. Most of the games utilize both the hemispheres of the brain.

Mahjong is a very popular game in the Far East. Playing mahjong can help seniors improve cognitive activities. Mahjong is a good game because it requires people to make fast decisions, analyze problems in new ways. It is a social game as well. It is taxing on Alzheimer's since it is a difficult game.

Crossword puzzle improves vocabulary, concentration, and memory. Can improve word fluency. Word search improves vocabulary. Good fund of vocabulary aids conversation and socialization. Overall board games are good to improve eye-hand coordination, improving abilities to use strategies and above all is good for socialization. Social interactions protect against cognitive deterioration, keeps one alert and active. Socializing maintains brain health as well as physical and mental.

Jigsaw puzzle is beneficial for cognitive development and character building. It teaches patience and perseverance. Jigsaw puzzles can teach problem-solving, project management skills, self-management skills, visuo spatial, tactile and social skills.

Sudoku is popular with seniors. Colorku is the color Sudoku Puzzle. Colorful wooden balls are used instead of numbers to solve puzzle. Colorku enhances visual processing, logic, reasoning, problem-solving strategies and problem-solving skills.

SET is a visual perception game which uses the left and right brain. Creativity requires the use of both the left and right sides of the brain.

Rail Road Rush Hour is a puzzle that demands attention, concentration, sequential thinking, visual problem-solving, critical thinking, and logic, reasoning and strategy development.

Seniors who live alone find crafts and puzzles as enjoyable pastime besides improving cognitive abilities. Crafts and puzzles exercise fingers and hands. Craft activities improve tactile sensation as well. Being involved with enjoyable activities keep one psychologically healthy and keeps depression at bay. Most of these puzzles are ideal to train early Alzheimer's and keep seniors engaged in intellectual activities.

Keeping occupied and stimulated can improve quality of life for the persons with dementia, as well as for those around them.

Activities can act as an opportunity for fun and playfulness. They also encourage independence, social inclusion, communication and expression of feelings.

In USA and England, many colleges and universities have lifelong learning programs taught by professors. In India, classes for variety of activities are conducted by private parties for a price.

A country as diverse as India is symbolized by the plurality of its culture. India has one of the world's largest collections of songs, music, folk dances, and classical dances, theatres, folk traditions, performing arts, rites and rituals, paintings and writings that are known as the "Intangible Cultural Heritage (ICH) of Humanity".

Drawing, painting, knitting, music, woodworking, playing games and solving puzzles are excellent cognitive activities for older seniors and these activities can be modified for early Alzheimer's.

Women in India are engaged in activities in arts and crafts, like embroidery, knitting, sewing, ceramics, beading, jewellery, painting, gourmet cooking, making different types of savouries, medley of sweets, pickles, curry masalas, gardening, making strands of jasmine flowers in the evening to make offering to the deity, or adorn one's hair. The mild-moderate ADIs should be encouraged to practice folk dances, folk art and music. Some usual activities for both men and women are flower arrangements, bird watching, and study creatures in the wild. Watching fish of many hues, and shapes swimming frolically in the fish tank, or in a pond is enjoyable and is relaxing. Learn about different herbs. Herbs are a great indoor-garden choice because they offer several kinds of sensory stimulation; the strong scents and tastes of the herbs, their medicinal value, the feel of the soil, and the bright colours of the leaves of some herbs. Some of the other activities are garden designing, restoring second hand furniture, placing indoor plants like spider plants, orchids in bathrooms.

There are many types of activities that maintain and improve the cognitive skills of older seniors and people who are victims of Alzheimer's disease.

Refer to Easy Craft Ideas by Pinterest. Pinterest gives manifold ideas as to how to paint glass, clay pots, pumpkins and gourds and much more. Each activity is explained in detail. The 'Hand painting wine glasses or plain glasses' instruction is given in detail step by step, from the beginning to the finish. It even gives details about the paints and brush to use. Activities are chosen depending on the ADs interest and abilities.

Take part in outdoor activity like fishing, bird watching, and be amazed about the century-old sandalwood tree and delicate wild flowers sprinkled with morning dew and animals in their natural habitat. Involve nature in treatment. A US study found that people who walked around an arboretum did 20 per cent better on a memory test than those who walked around the streets. Just looking at pictures of nature can have a beneficial effect.

"To the eyes of man of imagination, Nature is imagination itself." (William Blake)

"Keep a green tree in your heart and perhaps a singing bird will come." (Chinese proverb)

Involvement of children in adult activities may help seniors learn new things besides feeling younger and energetic. Conversation with younger family members can have a positive impact on the well-being of the person with dementia. Get them engaged in expressing themselves about their past interests like books, sports and other events. Take field trips to a place in the outskirts of a city for a picnic that would be good to reminisce of the past. People with dementia can often remember the distant past more easily than recent events. Activities focusing on reminiscence can help improve mood and well-being. They promote social inclusion and seeing the person as an individual with a unique life experience. It is a good way of helping relatives and friends stay connected. Above all, ADIs need a regular change of scenery, stimulation of fresh air and the outdoor environment.

Cardiorespiratory endurance (aerobic) activity, can benefit older people. Stronger muscles reduce the risk of falling and improve the ability to help perform the routine tasks. Among adults aged 65 years and older, walking and gardening or yard work are, by far, the most popular physical activities.

Another option includes a visit to a shopping mall or a theatre show, attend carnatic music recital, Bharatanatyam in sculpturesque poses, and attend a sporting event at a stadium. Utilize all the community facilities that accord joy and social interactions. Just because they are old and may suffer from early Alzheimer's doesn't mean that they wouldn't like to attend all the above events and to go window shopping or watch sports.

Intellectuals who suffer from mild to moderate Alzheimer's may be interested in the study of forts in India, temples, mosques and churches in India. They are educationally inspiring, while architecturally enchanting. Some people are still interested in collecting stamps, coins, postcards, and things of interest. Those interested in these activities can share information and converse on them.

Other activities for ADIs are: Sing old songs, make bird cages, feed birds and animals. Encourage ADIs to talk about their past interests and activities. Involve them to talk about current events, discoveries and inventions. Encourage them to talk about flags of different countries. Play intellectual games with the help of others if need be. The activities are varied but choose the activities that the ADI is familiar—with and interested in. An occupational therapist will be of help to choose activities for the dementia patients. The brain can indeed continue to renew itself, especially the hippocampus area that affects memory. Mild to moderate Alzheimer's are likely to follow instructions to complete an activity. However, instructions must be simple and given in steps depending on the level of comprehension.

Music Therapy (MT): Musical memory is often retained when other memories are lost. There are many ways to enjoy music, including listening, singing, following the rhythm and moving to the music. Evidence suggests that music can improve someone's mood, behavior and well-being. Studies have shown differences in brain plasticity due to stimulation of learning or practicing a musical instrument. The various elements of music are processed in the prefrontal cortex of the brain. Emotional memories that evoke emotions such as love and affection are very often well preserved for patients with Alzheimer's disease (Wikipedia). In the Music and Memory website Oliver Sacks, M.D. Professor and researcher of Columbia University, stated at "Having severe dementia means one can remember very little of one's past. But one will always remember familiar songs that one has listened to and sung." Hogeway in Netherlands has all the amenities that a human being wants. The residents are advanced Alzheimer's patients but lead a normal life within the confines of this village for Alzheimer's. "If you are demented a patient said, demented person does not have to sit alone." Music is very much encouraged at Hogeway. An Alzheimer's patient who has severe memory problems sang when her husband played the piano.

An interview with Dr. Julene Johnson, PhD, UCSF an expert on dementia and music when interviewed: "Are patients suffering from Alzheimer's disease able to retain memory of music while losing other essential and important cognitive function? Yes. It looks like that is true. They are pretty good in remembering familiar music."

Maestro Eduardo Marturet who is a composer, music director and conductor of the Miami Symphony Orchestra states: "Playing a musical instrument improves memory since it stimulates almost all the parts of the brain. Music and memory go hand in hand. Music at an early age can help improve a child's learning ability and memory" (Wikipedia). He reiterates this point when he says, "Further research has shown that participation in music at an early age can help improve a child's learning ability and memory. Music education is also linked to higher IQ levels and the development of certain parts of the brain. Furthermore he states that music relieves stress, makes one smarter, improves social life, and improves confidence, patience, and discipline. Music fosters creativity and improves memory." In south India Classical music and classical dances are culturally embedded in the lives of children and their parents. It is common knowledge that these art forms improve intelligence, memory and specially math abilities.

Helpful suggestions to improve concentration and memory of Alzheimer's:

1. Choose an activity that ADIs are interested in and want to complete. In order to retain memory, concentrate on the activity at hand even if it is simple. Reduce distractions for efficient learning. The more one exercises the brain on a subject, the better the memory for that activity. Over learn.
2. Involve as many senses as possible specially visual and auditory. Try to relate information to colors, textures, smells, and tastes. The physical act of revising information can help imprint it in the brain. Even if you're a visual learner, read out loud what you want to remember. If you can recite it rhythmically, it is even better.
3. Discard faulty information processing so that it does not interfere with new knowledge. It is prudent for the ADIs to assimilate new ideas more with ease into what they already know. It is judicious to start with simple games like Chinese checkers, snakes and ladders for ADIs instead of Sudoku and Chess which are strategy games. In sewing select simple patterns so that ADIs can accomplish the task. If anybody wants to practice cooking, choose a recipe that is simple and very familiar. Food recipes are available on the Internet and participants can share these ideas or they can share their grandma's recipes. Besides engaging in this social event, one can learn and remember ideas about cooking. People can help each other on several practical persuasions while learning new ideas and remembering them. Cooking is one of the best pastime for people these days.

   There is an abundance of games on the Internet and most of them while are entertaining are very helpful to stimulate the brain; to concentrate, learn, relearn and remember (Refer to: Memory-Improvement_Tips. com.) For instance, the Bubble hit-Bubble Breaker game improves concentration and is fun. Cambridge Brain sciences has a new test. This test deals with memory, reasoning, concentration and planning. It is more like Luminosity. These tests may be too hard for ADIs but are cognitively stimulating to the intelligent people. For a full-brain workout, play a variety of games often. Different games strengthen different mental abilities. Some of these games should keep intelligence in constant repair. Most of these games are based on WAIS 1V and V, and WMS 1V and V.

4. *Organize information.* How can you remember a phone number 86421357? Learn in groups like 8642 (shows difference of two in descending order and 1357 in ascending order). Chunking method is helpful. Chunking is especially helpful for remembering long sequences of numbers such as phone and account numbers 10 to 12 digits long or more. In order to remember new information, summarize the information. Organized information is easier to retain than random information. Visualizing information that has been read are retained better. Alzheimer's have to adopt simple methods to organize.
5. *Use mnemonics.* That is, tie information to visual images, sentences, acronyms, or rhymes. An example of rhyme or poem mnemonics is, "Thirty days hath September, April, June and November; All the rest have thirty-one, save February, with twenty-eight days clear, and twenty-nine each leap year."
6. *Rehearse information.* Maintenance rehearsal is the process of repeatedly verbalizing or thinking about a piece of information. Disrupting rehearsal is not very effective for encoding long-term memory. Elaborative rehearsal like organizing, thinking about, and linking new material to existing memories is more effective. Encoding by meaning, encoding by images, encoding

by organization are better remembered. More the associations, the more the cues for retrieval. Teach what you learned to another person to improve memory. Overlearn/overdo to reduce memory interference. Meditation, visualization and association create strong memory links.

7. Distributing learning decreases the rate of forgetting compared to mass learning and enhances memory consolidation. ADIs get easily distracted and frustrated and thus any new activity will have to be distributed over time. (In teaching any one playing card game, explain the game in simple language and step by step.) Gradually. introduce different types of card games before attempting to introduce them to Bridge. Gradually, teach them all the techniques used in bidding and playing. Do not force people to play difficult card games.
8. The more one exercises the mind on a theme/activity, the better the memory for that activity. This method can be used to teach any activity, including cooking, crafts, art, budgeting, keeping accounts, taking care of oneself and so on.
9. *Develop a healthy lifestyle.* Be committed to healthy diet, take regular exercise have happy thoughts and have good friends. Avoid smoking and avoid excessive drinking of alcohol.
10. Sleep is necessary for memory consolidation; alertness, and for focussed attention and concentration. Deep sleep is good for learning and memory.
    a. Learning strengthened by later-stage sleep. Spindle-rich sleep that occurs in the latter half of a night's sleep is responsible for strengthened learning ability.
    b. Sleep reorganizes memories and improves creativity. Research suggests that sleep reorganizes and restructures memories, and identify the most important details.

c. Sleep strengthens memories, protects from interference. Non-distracted participants who slept after learning 20 word pairs recalled 12 per cent more. (They are normal adults.)

Cognitive training decreases risk of cognitive decline. This 800-page research study, funded by the National Institutes of Health (NIH) USA, recommends strategies to improve memory. Training to improve cognitive abilities in older people lasted to some degree 10 years after the training program was completed, according to results of a randomized clinical trial supported by the National Institutes of Health. The findings showed training improved cognition involved in the ability to think and learn. Spacing of practice influences training and transfer. Overlearn the material that will be useful in life. Dementia patients need several repetitions of an activity in order to preserve the memory for that specific activity. Memory exercise increases hippocampus size and improves memory. Short 20-minute concentration meditation can improve concentration.

There are numerous games to improve memory and thinking, sensory perception, coordination/motor skills, critical thinking and problem-solving. Toy stores have games that incorporate the principles underlying neuropsychological tests.

Memory guru of India: This is more likely for those who have normal intelligence and memory who want to better their cognitive abilities.

Online brain-training: Does it really work? Those who are interested may refer to an article online brain-training: "Does it Really Work?" by Elizabeth Day, *The Observer*, Sunday, 21 April 2013: "I find they are interesting to play and can transfer to other situations akin to one I have been playing. For instance for matching test, all I needed was good concentration. Intelligent people will find these tests interesting and people with Alzheimer's may improve their cognitive abilities. These tests are very expensive, compared to video games."

There are fun games on the Internet for children and adults who want to have a diversion from serious work.

Strategies for Cognitive Stimulation

Attention, concentration and tracking and ways to improve cognition through training using the following methods.

Visual Search and Attention Test (VSAT) to cross out letters and symbols that are identical to a target.

The Span Tests

The Span Tests come in the format of number of digits, amount of information retained by a person to immediately report regarding what is seen and what is heard. Attention Span Test, 10 questions, five min. is a test for attention deficit and distractibility. How long can one focus on a task without getting distracted.

Digit Span

This is to repeat digits heard for example 264 forward and backward.

Tests like Knox Cube Test Revised: Measures short-term memory and attention span. Is useful in identification of ADD. Any block test can be used to train ADIs.

Dot Location Task

This consists of dots up to nine on a sheet of paper. The S is instructed to repeat the drawing of the dots in the same order of presentation.

Sentence Repetition

Repeat sentences that are administered.

Mental Tracking

The simplest test is to make a person to repeat digits backwards. This utilizes perceptual tracking and more complex operations. Another test is Speech Sound Perceptual Test. The subject has to pay constant attention. This is to train ADIs to discriminate like and unlike pairs of musical beats. Simple example is to tap say four times on the desk and vary the number of taps and ask the ADIs to replicate the taps.

The Reversed Digit Span

Digits should be presented like 86371 and the ADI has to repeat the numbers in reverse order.

Serial Subtraction

Serial sevens, counting from one hundred by sevens is a clinical test and is difficult even for some clinicians. To improve concentration, train the ADIs with serial 3s. Even better is two which will be least stressful.

The Test of Sustained Attention and Tracking (TSAT)

This test includes two mental control items (alphabet and counting backwards from 20), serial subtraction of 3s from 100 to 70, plus days of the week and months of the year forward and backward plus asking for numbers and letters alternatively 1-A-2-B and so on. This trains sustained attention and concentration.

Alpha Span

This method trains short-term memory and mental tracking. The individual is asked to repeat eight unrelated words with instruction to repeat them in alphabetical order. For both young and old this test proved to be difficult at seven words. Research suggests that training can improve encoding and retrieval processes in the elderly, leading to better memory functioning. [Glisky, E.L. and Glisky, M.L. (1999), "Memory Rehabilitation in the Elderly"]

Paced Auditory Serial Addition Test (PASAT)

On giving "2-8-6-1-9" and when called out 8 the Subject (S) calculates the numbers as 10, 14, 7, 10. 8 (eight) is added to 2+10 and 8+6 is 14; 6+1+ 7 and 9+1 = 10. Each number is delivered at a speed of 1.2 seconds to 2.4 seconds but in case of ADI time is not a factor, but learning is. This test improves concentration and cognitive abilities. ADIs may be reluctant to engage in this test but once they start and with help they will learn to do this test. Is a good test to exercise concentration and memory.

Trail Making Test (TMT)

This test involves complex visual scanning with a motor component with motor speed and agility The Trail Making Test B monitors planning ability as well as visuo-motor speed, Visual scanning, visuo-spatial ability, mental flexibility, concentration, and executive functions.

1 8

5

3

7

4

6 2 9

Connect the numbers in serial order like 1 to 2 and 3 to 4 and so on. One can make it more complex. Place an alphabet to the numbers like 1a, 9i and so on. Visual representation may give more flexibility and speed of learning.

Symbol digit modalities:

Digit Symbol. The symbols are paired with digits 1 to 9 and the individual is directed to mark as many of the symbols that correspond to the digits within the prescribed time. This requires rapid eye movement, motor abilities and short-term visual memory.

1 = @ 2 = # 3 = $ 4 = &. Make up your own symbols for the numerals. This type of exercises improves attention span, visual scanning and motor speed. One has to find the symbol for 1 and so on.

Vigilance Test

In experiments, the subjects are asked to tap when a green light is shown and not to any other color lights. This trains in selective attention. In order to attain a driver's license, one has to take this test through the department of transportation. Simple way to train is "When I tap twice you lift your ring finger and not to any other taps."

The Digit Vigilance Test

The Digit Vigilance Test respondents are asked to find and cross out either sixes or nines, which appear randomly within 59 rows of single digits on two separate pages. This test can be administered to individuals with age range 20 to 80. This test can be modified to suit the ADIs. Can be modified to suit the AD individual.

Cancellation by using digits and letters in various combinations. This needs vigilance and speed, since it is a timed test. Exercises on this type of tests are meant to improve visuo-spatial abilities and thus can improve functions on ADLs. Train the individual to remember numbers by practicing. Auditory Digit Span can be used to train memory for numbers.

Show the map of your city and request ADIs to go to a particular town using a pencil and use the finger to show the direction. Training on such tests can improve sense of directions, routes and locations. People who tend to get lost can be trained on this test so that they can assess directions. It will be even better to map the surroundings of the home of the ADI and make the individual to take different routes at different time to a particular location.

Constructional Activities

Cloak drawing or any drawing in straight lines connecting them in a meaning full manner. This will improve directions, thinking and concentration. Lego is a popular line of construction toys manufactured by The Lego Group. It involves both right and left brains.

Orientation and Attention

Orientation to time, place and person. Alzheimer's have difficulty with orientation. Teach them to get used to calendars, watches, directions like east, west, north, and south. If necessary remind the person of time, place and person frequently if need be.

Test of Spatial Orientation

Draw a line and ask the person to close eyes and draw over the line. The following questions can be improvised to meet the needs of the subjects. Can you estimate the speed of the car ahead of you? Can you estimate the distance between your car and the car ahead of you? Place two objects on the table at a distance of a foot. Ask the patient to estimate the distance between the two objects. Play the Maze game and games of this order.

Left-Right Orientation

Make a pathway with left and right turns as in Maze test. Show a map with starting point and the destination with indications for left and right turns. Train the person in an activity like this, so that ADIs will have better orientation to the surroundings and directional sense.

Build three-dimensional block figures using front, top, and side views. Training on blocks can improve depth perception of objects. For instance, it helps ADIs to navigate around footsteps in the house or outside.

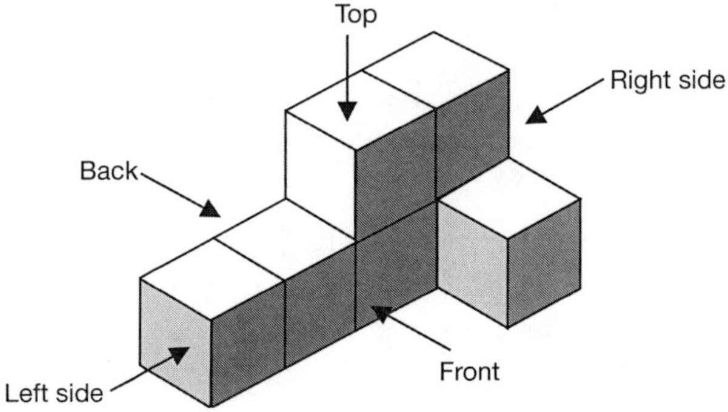

Figure: Three-Dimensional Structure: Direction of Views

Source: Internet google.com

How many blocks will you need to build the following:

These two shapes different? Or are they identical and merely oriented differently?

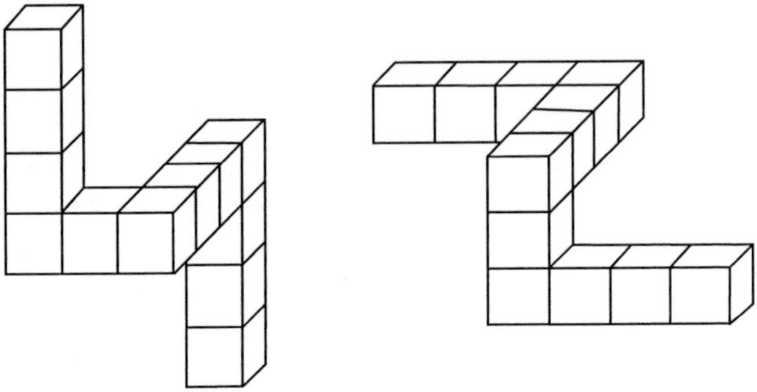

— Spatial intelligence in children by Gwen Dewar Ph.D.

Try building these. How many blocks are there?

See more at: http://www.parentingscience.com/spatial-intelligence.html#sthash.0HltXn3Q.dpufvvv

Temporal orientation: Ask the ADI as to the day of the week, day of the month, month, year and time of the day. Show different faces and label them. ADIs have to remember these faces when picture of faces are shown a second time and perhaps on other occasions.

Complete a picture that has been cut in parts. ADIs has to visualize the picture to put the parts together.

Everyone has to know basics of Arithmetic to balance the check book, buy groceries and so on. Train the ADIs with basics of math.

Present 75 63 41 and ask the person to do it in reverse order. Increase the length of the Digits till you find that the ADI is not able to concentrate. Do not force an individual to perform beyond his/her capacity. Some individuals may be able to go beyond even 4 numbers forwards and backwards. Example: 54372 forwards and 27345 backwards.

All arithmetical operations are necessary in our daily living. Thus make the ADI to practice on simple math.

Example: 4+2= 6–3= 3×3= 16 divided by 4=

8+3= 8–3= 5×5= 20 divided by 4=

Give pencil and paper to calculate higher numbers.

Example: 23+26= 40+52= 15×10= 21×18=

Ram has 32 apples and he gave the apples to four friends equally dividing the apples. How many did each one get?

The train is going at a speed of 50 miles an hour. How many hours will it take for the train to cover 500 miles?

Ice cream costs per cone 12 rupees. You want to buy 12 of them. How much will you give the ice cream vendor?

Administer Serial subtraction of 3 from 20 and then increase to higher numbers. For instance ask the AD to subtract 5 from 100. Trials should be demonstrated and do not push the patient but can be encouraged compassionately. These tests can be repeated to evaluate the improvement. Do not try serial Subtractions of 7 from 100. Many will find it very hard to do this. To train to maintain attention and concentration these tests can be modified to suit the ADI.

Continuous Additions

2-------------

3-------------5

5-------------8

7-------------12

The ADI is instructed by demonstration to add the successive overlapping pairs as fast as possible and to write the results on the right side of two adjoining vertical numbers. If the client feels exhausted, give a break.

Arithmetical Reasoning

How many are 4 and 8 oranges?

How many oranges are in 6 dozens?

A thermometer that reads 64 degrees goes up 6 degrees and then drops 7 degrees. What is the current reading?

2 pounds of fish cost ₹ 2 and 50 Paisa. How many pounds can you buy with ₹ 10.00?

At 50 miles an hour, how long would it take a car to go 100 miles?

A pound of cabbage costs 20 paisa, how many pounds could you get for 100 paisa?

Write down ₹ 10, 100, 1000, 10,000 and 100,000 and read out.

A. 56440, B. 56450, C. 56504, D. 45650 which is the lowest number.

Read the following numbers: 4780, 3892, 5643, and 7866. Pick out the highest number and the lowest.

Directions: Using 9, 0, 5, 2, four digits once only: compile your number.

Smallest Five Digit number is -----------

A. 20459 B. 40259 C. 02459 D. 50294

Largest 5 digit number is:

A. 95024 B. 95420 C. 90524 D. 94520

Write down the highest to the lowest values

A. 8734; 82541; 9012; 9749

Find the value of: 84149 – 22611=

Man bought 10 boxes of canned mango juice for a party. There were 12 cans in each box. How many cans of mango did he buy in total?

Anil bought 4 packets of chocolates and 6 packets of M@M. Each packet contained 10 of each. In total how many chocolates and M&M.

A Thermometer that reads 61 degrees goes up 9 degrees and then drops 2 degrees. What does it read then?

Three men can clear a blocked road in 35 minutes; how many can clear it in 14 minutes or less?

Numerals and Alphabet

Average rate for reading assorted letters and alphabet is, at grade school graduation is over two and half letters per second. But on further education speed will be much higher. But in cases of ADIs we have to be patient and let the patient go at the speed one chooses. Case letters lower and higher have different speeds. ADIs may be confused a bit and so be patient. This is to help them and not to enter for an examination.

6183904725; 85629310428 and so on. Give several sets of numbers in order to encourage patient to read.

Now alphabets: from A to Z (a to z)

A k l s m k r h u j z o b t d w I m y r a h q n p e u. Give more of alphabets to read till the patient is able to read faster.

Now try this. A1 b2 c3 4d 5e; 6ab 7cd 8ef 9gh 10ij

Now Alphabet in upper case:

A B C D E F G H I J K L M N O P Q R S T U V W X Y Z.

K Q V D A W B S E L G C M U F Y R N Z P T I X O J H

P G F R J O L N V X O L D S A M K D

Tests on Vocabulary

This is to encourage patient to use words that are familiar and a few unfamiliar. This helps patient to use words to communicate with others.

Stanford-Binet Intelligence Scale contains several words.

> water, cup, sister, walk, butter, crowd, indict, learn, take power, fan, box, hot, her, his, we, get, jug, peon, odor, nosy, noisy, horse, elephant, church, temple, mosque, void, wind, which, wash, whim, wipe, wire

Use words that are simple if the patient is in the moderate stage of AD.

Best word club offers 4-letter word ending in E

www.bestwordclub.com/en/wl/4letterwordsendingine.htm

List of four-letter words ending with E. abbe, able, abye, ache, acme, acne, acre, adze, agee, ague, aide, aine, ajee, akee, alae, albe, alee, alme, aloe, amie, ance, ...

Letter word ending in C

Exec • Fisc • Flic • Floc • Huic...

www.bestwordclub.com/en/wl/4letterwordsendinginc.htm

One word ending in C and O. Word finder.

> List of four-letter words ending with C. abac, aesc, alec, atoc, banc, bloc, chic, choc, croc, disc, douc, drac, emic, epic, eric, etic, exec, fisc, flic, floc, fusc, huic, laic, ...

www.bestwordclub.com/en/wl/4letterwordsendingino.htm

> List of four-letter words ending with O. aero, afro, agio, alco, alko, also, alto, ambo, ammo, anno, apso, arco, arvo, auto, bego, biro, bito, boho, boko, bolo, boyo, ...

Poem Reading: some already have their favorite poems. The members can read out loud for the rest of them and have a discussion on it.

Indians like to sing Bajans, songs of their movie stars, classical music. Most people enjoy classical music. Keep a time table for different activities and make music as one of the favorite activity. Even people who don't sing may join a chorus. Rhythmic type songs also may be introduced since some may get up and dance to the tune. Western countries people dance to a tune whereas majority of Indians rather sit and chat than dare an activity like dancing to a tune. We can always try. After the initial hesitation, if a few people get up to dance, others may follow.

Arrange an occasion to narrate enjoyable anecdotes.

Opposites or Antonyms

Admit (deny), Advantage (Disadvantage) agree (disagree), Black (White)

Blame (praise), Brave (cowardly), deep-(shallow), honest (dishonest)

Inferior (superior)

Complimentary antonyms are word pairs that have no degree of meaning. There are only two opposite possibilities.

Dead – alive; True – false; Male – female; Daughter – son; On – off

Disorders of reading attributed to strephosymbolia are manifested in large part by reading exposed material from right to left. Read the following words in opposite direction.

ON PIN LIVE NOT PAN DOOR BUT LAP ROOM WAS RAT

- Racecar, peep
- Stressed or desserts
- Rewarder or redrawer
- Departer or retraped
- Stop or pots
- Snap or pans
- Star or rats
- Diaper or repaid

Encourage the patients to communicate with familiar words. Cognitive therapy will work with mild to moderate ADIs.

The longest known palindrome in the Oxford Dictionary is “tattarrattat”. The longest palindrome in use today is said to be the Finnish word "saippuakivikauppias" which means soap stone vendor. A derivative of this is the palindrome "saippuakalasalakauppias" meaning soapfish bootlegger.

Encourage the patients to communicate with familiar words. Cognitive therapy will work with mild to moderate ADIs.

TOP TAP NOW NOD RAIL TIDE TEN
TIME DEER WAR PART

NO NIP EVIL TON DON EDIT TUB
NAP ROOD ERA PIT MOOR

Differences and Likenesses

The patient has to explain the differences and likenesses of the given pairs. The answers are rated depending on the merit of the answers. However, the attempt here is to encourage patients to think and remember the meaning of familiar words and how to use them appropriately.

Aberration - alteration

Anomaly - antithesis

Departure - deviation

Objection - opposition

Nonacceptance - noncompliance

Do these words confuse you?

Accede - exceed	adapt - adept - adopt
addition - edition	Aloud - allowed
allusion - illusion	appraise - apprise

Explain the following concepts

***Examples*:**

Bread	made of flour	food
House	Built out of wood	buildings

Knife	use them to eat or cut with	eating, utensils
Pencil	To write with them	things to write with
Room	belong to the house	parts of the house
Watch	Tell time	clock
Axe	Cut with them	Tools

(refer to Illustration Concepts by Pinterest)

Differences between

Bread and cakes

House and Villa

Knife and spoon

Pencil and Pen

Room and balcony

Watch and clock

Axe and Saw

Day and night

Word Association

These word lists are based on either Jung or Kent. For trials the following words may be used. Apple; tree; knife; fresh; driver.

Instruction: I am going to read you a list of ordinary English words, one by one, and each time I give you a word answer with the first word that comes to your mind when you hear the word I speak. Let us try one or two words for practice.

> Girl, Rose, time, garden, window, apple, woman, ship, run, fish, mother, brother, friend, school, teacher, drama, dance

Sentence Building

Since we are training ADIs, while administering this test, give attention to difficulty formulating a grammatical sentence. As long as the patient can build a sentence conveying meaning, it may be accepted but note the grammatical mistakes.

Correct the following sentences:

Kent has given examples of faulty sentences that score 0. "The hunter has a dog - he hunts for wolves." "The automobile had a flat in the tire so they had a delay."

Instruction: Build sentences using the following words.

Broom--------------woman------------floor

Corner-------------car------------------man

Child---------------play----------------toy

Mother-------------cooking------------kitchen

Delay---------------tire------------------automobile

House--------------girl------------------bird

Lake----------------stick----------------dog

Narrate your feelings about your caregiver in a few sentences to another patient. Allow the other patient to tell her/his feelings and experiences of the day with the caregiver.

Absured Sentences

Absurd means: what is foolish, does not make sense unreasonable, illogical.

ADIs may not be able to give correct answers. Therefore, instead of correcting, encourage them to think logically step by step.

- *ICE*: They put it on the stove instead of in the icebox.

  You will not put it on the stove because it will melt all the more.

  It won't keep it from melting if you put it on the stove.
- *RAIN*: Two weeks could not come that fast, it takes fourteen days and here it says it took only one day. If it rained yesterday, it couldn't be two weeks; it would be just the day after.

  You may give any number of words to the patient as long as the patient is interested in continuing with the test.

Normal Limits of Answers

To make the test more interesting two meaningful words can be given as follows:

- *Winter-Leaves*: Leaves on the trees, and there aren't in winter. No leaves in late winter, it would be fall. Not many colors, colors in the fall.
- *Hunter-Birds*: You don't shoot with an axe. A hunter does not carry an axe; he carries a gun.
- *Dusty-Rain*: The road will be all wet. Rain will make it muddy and dirty.
- *Hammer-Bolt*: It would not turn a hammer, you will bang it; a bolt is a screw anyway, not a nail.
- *Silver-Lead-Gold*: It does matter whether gold is more valuable than either.

  How would you know if silver is more valuable than lead just because gold is valuable.
- *Rock-Tree*: If he was walking toward the tree he was walking forward and would not bump the back of his head unless walking backward. He could not hit a tree if he was away from it; back of head cannot hit a tree if you are walking forward.
- Other examples are Deers-wolves; thunder-lightning. You can make your own to suit the abilities of your patient.

The football was blown up so hard that, when it fell in the water, it sank.

It was four O'clock in the evening and by running as he thought he could get home by 1 O'clock.

The man put heavy stones in the boat, so that it would not move so deep in the water.

It takes a man thirty minutes to walk to the village, but three men can walk there in ten minutes.

Absurdities to Laugh About

"I want to write my own eulogy, and I want to write it in Latin. It seems only fitting to read a dead language at my funeral." —Jarod Kintz, *I Want*

Attorney Jokes: Attorney: Were you present when your picture was taken?

Witness: You are kidding me, right?

Two boys go for a walk. One of them says: let me walk in the middle.

For money we can even work free.

Mirror is my best friend, because when I cry it does not laugh.

What are you doing? Wife said, I lost my brain. I am looking for it.

Simple Sentences to Repeat

Maya gave her daughter a bicycle for her birthday last week

At two clock tomorrow he will be giving a lecture.

I gave my daughter an airline ticket to go to London for her birthday. She will visit the Buckingham Palace and tower of London.

Anil's mother gave him a ticket to go to the cricket match.

Be sure to make them sing because it will improve speech.

Sentence repetition: Direct the person to repeat after you from very simple sentence to a sentence with 10 words.

Can the person repeat 4th grade rhyming poetry. Simplest level may be "Jack and Jill went up the hill" and "Baba black sheep". Learn the following poem and repeat.

1. Up! up! my Friend, and quit your books;
   Or surely you'll grow double: (fir time pass kar lo thori der may tea ka time honey wala)
   Up! up! my Friend, and clear your books;
   Why all this toil and trouble? (by Wordsworth)

2. I love snow and all the forms
   Of the radiant frost, I love waves and winds and storms
   Everything almost which is Nature's and may be
   Untainted by man's misery.

(by Percy Bysshe Shelley)

Select a short poem in the language of the ADI to learn and to repeat.

Let the ADIs narrate their own stories. Make them remember the stories and poems from first grade.

Make them narrate childhood experiences. Narrate fables: and ask questions on them in order to assess comprehension and memory. In this case, it will be immediate memory.

Fables: The Wolf in Sheep's Clothing

One day a wolf found a sheepskin. He covered himself with the sheepskin and got into a flock of sheep grazing in a field. He thought, "The shepherd will shut the sheep in the pen after sunset. At night I will run away with a fat sheep and eat it."

All went well till the shepherd shut the sheep in the pen and left. The wolf waited patiently for the night to advance and grow darker. But then an unexpected thing happened. One of the servants of the shepherd entered the pen. His master had sent him to bring a fat sheep for supper. The servant picked up the wolf dressed in the sheepskin.

That night the shepherd and his guests had the wolf for supper.

Moral: An evil design has an evil end.

The Ant and the Grasshopper

On a summer day, a merry grasshopper was dancing, singing and playing his violin with all his heart. He saw an ant passing by, bearing along with great toil a wheat ear to store for the winter.

"Come and sing with me instead of working so hard", said the grasshopper, "Let's have fun together."

"I must store food for the winter", said the ant, "and I advise you to do the same."

"Don't worry about winter, it's still very far away", said the grasshopper, laughing at him. But the ant wouldn't listen and continued his toil.

When the winter came, the starving grasshopper went to the ant's house and humbly begged for something to eat.

"If you had listened to my advice in the summer you would not now be in need", said the ant. "I'm afraid you will have to go to bed without supper" and he closed the door.

Moral of the story is: "It is best to prepare for the days of necessity."

One day a man was going to the market with his son and his donkey. They met a couple on the way. "Why walk when you have a donkey to ride" called out the husband. "Seat the boy on the donkey" I would like that said the boy and asked his father to help him to mount the donkey. Soon they met another couple and the woman said "let your father ride". Now the donkey has two riders. Then, one of the travelers cried out "How cruel of them. They are going to kill the donkey." Hearing this father and son got down and decided to carry the donkey on their shoulders. The travelers broke into laughter which frightened the donkey. It broke free and galloped away.

Proverbs are given to find out the ability for abstraction. These days hardly any one uses proverbs. However, if you want to use proverbs to assess abstraction, administer them taking into account the language of the person. In India people speak different languages and use proverbs that are culture centered.

English proverbs are familiar to educated classes in India. Instruction to be given is as follows:

I will explain the proverb, you tell me the proverb.

> Milk: after it happens, forget it (Do not cry over spilt milk)

In Hindi it is: "Ab Pachhtaaye hote kya, jab chidiya chug gayi khet?" Translation "What is the use of crying when the birds ate the whole farm."

> *Dog*: Loud mouthed people do not amount much. (Barking dogs seldom bite)
>
> *Wheel*: If you want to get something, you better let people know about (squeaky wheels get the grease).
>
> *Door*: Golden hammer is truth; truth will break away lies. (A golden hammer breaks iron door).

Explain the following:

One swallow does not make a summer.

The grass is always greener on the other side of the mountain

Still waters run deep.

Some Indian Proverbs: Bandar kya jaane adark ka swaad. (What does a monkey know the taste of ginger? Meaning: Someone without refined tastes cannot appreciate a fine thing.) English equivalent: Laying pearls before the swine.

Finishing sentences from prompts can feel good, and using well-worn adages that are deeply embedded in memory makes it easy.

Start by bringing up a complete old saying:

Seen but not---------------- (heard)

A stitch in time------------ (saves nine)

General Knowledge Test: Name the longest river in India.

India has the largest deposit of ____________ in the world. Choose: Gold, copper, mica* and none of the above.

What does Milkha Singh known for?

Where is the Satellite launching station in India (Sriharikotta, AP)

Who is the first Indian to go into space (Squadron Leader Rakesh Sharma)

Name a few snakes of India.

Tell me the names of a few Indian sweets.

What metal does a magnet attract?

What are the colors of the Indian National flag?

What is the capital of India?

How is the cloud formed?

Make the questions simpler to adapt to the patient. For instance, one can ask: name three spices that are used to cook meat or three spices that you generally use.

What are the precautions you will have to take against mosquito bites and why?

Do you know about purification of water? What type of water do you drink?

Do you want to talk on topics on hygiene?

Do you have phone numbers of hospital emergency unit?

Do you know your own phone number and address?

Answer each question the best you can.

How is a stone different from a tree?

How are the following different from each other?

Table-chair

Bird-Dog

Daisy-Rose

Dog-wolf

How is cotton used?

What is salt used for?

What do you do with a comb?

Ask for the meaning of simple words that are used every day.

What is the difference between dictionaries and encyclopedia

Some of the following items are taken from Wechsler-Bellevue Intelligence Scale:

In what way are the following alike?

Coat-dress;

Dog-Lion:

Daily News Paper-TV;

Air-water;

Bad-good

How many days are there in a week?

Who discovered America?

Who was Mahatma Gandhi?

Cup is to coffee as bowl is to: a. dish, b.*Soup, c. spoon d. food.

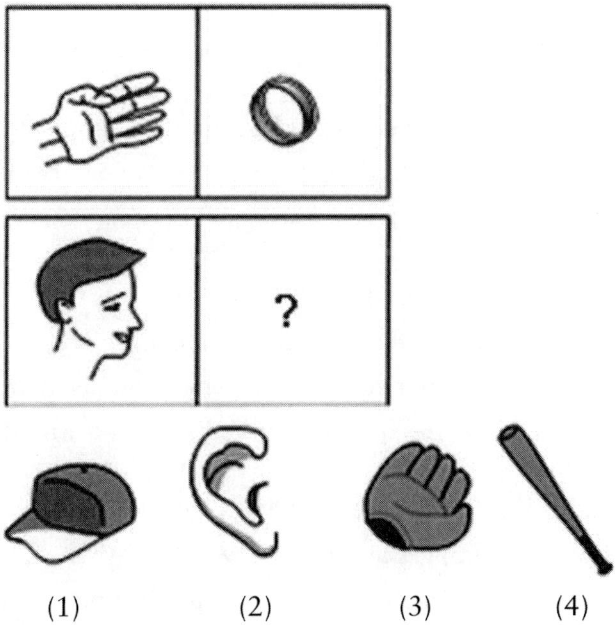

Source: India BIX.

Terms for group of animals:

Term used for lot of elephants----------------herd.

Term used for ants---------------------------A colony (army, swarm) of ants.

Term used for apes------------------------A troop of apes.

Birds------------------------------------A flock or parcel of birds.

Chicken-------------------------------- A brood, clutch, flock.

Collective noun for flowers----------------A bouquet of flowers, a bunch of flowers, a garden of flowers.

The Indian Institute of Science is located where? (Bengaluru)

Bagh village is famous for what? (Cave Painting)

Which city in India known as "Electronic city"? (Bengaluru)

In which state of India is Fort St. George? (Chennai)

Where is New York? (USA)

What is Ramayana? (Epic)

The place in North East India which receives the highest annual rainfall (Chirrapunji)

The industry for which Visakhapatnam is famous for?

What is the thing to do if there is fire in your home? Is it fire proof?

Why should we lock the door in the night?

What are the duties of the police?

What will you do if you are lost in a mall?

What will you do if you cut your finger by mistake?

Will you open the door for strangers if you are alone at home?

What is the other name for Bengaluru?

How many oranges are there in two dozens?

How much change will you get from 20 rupees when you pay only 11 rupees for the oranges?

Color Naming

Present a sheet on which different circled colors are presented in several lines. The patients have to name the colors as fast as they can. Although this test is used for various purposes, when administered to ADIs the examiner better not penalize the patient for mistakes or time taken. After all, this test also measures the time taken, confusion, tendency to make mistakes, difficulty in naming the colors, impatience and so forth. This test helps patients to concentrate, to think and remember. Over a period of time there will be a change in patient's performance. Practice makes one learn and remember.

Give a sample: Blue red yellow purple.

Present then a sheet of paper with various colors to be named.

A few of these items or the format is taken from a handbook I possess published by Psychological Corporation in 1945 but the publisher does not exist anymore.

Memory Span for Objects: When 20 objects are presented, an adult with normal intelligence will recall 11 objects and above. ADIs will be able to remember a few of them on repeated presentation of the objects. Use familiar objects with ADIs to reduce their frustration. People under stress do not learn well.

Flower, plant, rose, lily, jasmine, home, window, and door. Add more concepts if needed and words familiar to patients. Or request the ADIs to suggest five familiar objects and if need be reduce to three. Present them as pictures.

The objects must be familiar to patients and must be culled out from their experiences. Supplement these pictures from available places.

Show pictures of banana, mangoes, papaya, beat root and ask for similarities. This helps the person to talk about the uses of these fruits and associate them with their experiences. Papaya and bananas can be used as face mask to improve complexion. Ask for similarities among tea, coffee, coco, chocolate, coke.

Picture Similarities: Present pictures of vegetables and fruits. Ask for the similarities of them. "What is alike about them." Present tools, utensils, geometrical figures. Choose additional concepts that the ADIs may like. Make the ADIs to draw some of the geometric figures to improve the parietal lobe. It may even improve sense of directions in patients.

Name these fruits and their uses. Make the clients to talk about the following. They may free associate and tell stories. One way to make them communicate and use language. They may share recipes. Present a bunch of grapes, oranges, tomatoes and a display of several vegetables and ask for names and uses and their experience with them.

Show a picture of several familiar things and allow the patient to repeat as many as possible. How many of them can one remember after it is removed from view?

Name the following kitchen utensils and how they are used. Make a meal using these utensils.

Name all of them and when did you use them. How many of them can one remember after five minutes exposure? Present a jug, tea pot, coffee pot, cup and saucer, wine glass, campagne glass, glass used for water to drink, knife, fork, spoon, whisker, spatuala, roller pin, mixie, food processor and ask to remember some of them and utility. These will help them to visualize items and connect them to usage.

Indulge in enjoyable recollection of past experiences of childhood with your friends and relatives. Remember your childhood friends, your teachers, social events and reminisce about good times. Recite poems you learned. Sing along with the people you mix with or sing at home, have Fun with odd jokes but clean ones. "A child asked me why did the orange stop running?" then he answered "It ran out of juice." How do you kill a yellow elephant? "Who has ever heard of a yellow elephant?" Jokes improve socialization and mood. Talk about hilarious social events that you have experienced, to persuade the rest to join in relating their experiences, and enjoy laughing together.

Picture Absurdities: Like a cat in a cobweb; a cock with three legs, clothes on cloth line moving westward when the tree leaves are moving eastward.

For fun read "Jabberwocky" (disambiguation). "Jabberwocky" is considered one of the greatest nonsense poems written in English. It's playful, whimsical language has given

English nonsense words and neologisms such as Galumphing and Chortie.

Present Pictures with Absurdities: This exercise will train the brain to reason regarding the absurdities of the pictures. Each picture depicts meaningless state. The more the patient thinks and reasons, the better is the cognitive stimulation for the brain.

- *Example*: Regarding the picture of the two weights on one side and none on the other, the answer should be "This one (pointing to the weights) supposed to be heavier than that."
- *Snail*: Supposed to be a snail, his feet are not right. Rat got no snail back. Has three legs, should have two. (This is a picture with a snail on the back of a rat.)

Picture Discrimination: This test trains higher level of reasoning and judgment. The first picture which is a radio looks like a book, a flash light like a fountain pen, a Barometer like a clock.

Objects represented twice: Present picture cards that may elicit attention, grasp, comparison, discrimination, abstracting, judgment and reasoning. These pictures train the brain to reason and solve problems. These type of activities, assess several neuropsychological functions of attention, grasp, comparison, discrimination, abstraction, judgment, and reasoning.

Geometrical cross out test is a difficult one. Same geometric figures to be cancelled when other figures are included.

Picture Interpretation: The ADI person has to give the details of the picture, the scenario, the actions, interpretations and so on which is logical and meaningful. This test measures, comprehension, grasp, understanding and reasoning.

When presented with an activity like cooking say: Remember these fruits and vegetables. Direct people to make dishes that they fancy and share.

Present pictures in color to help them to remember better. Allow them to read out the items out loud. These factors will improve memory.

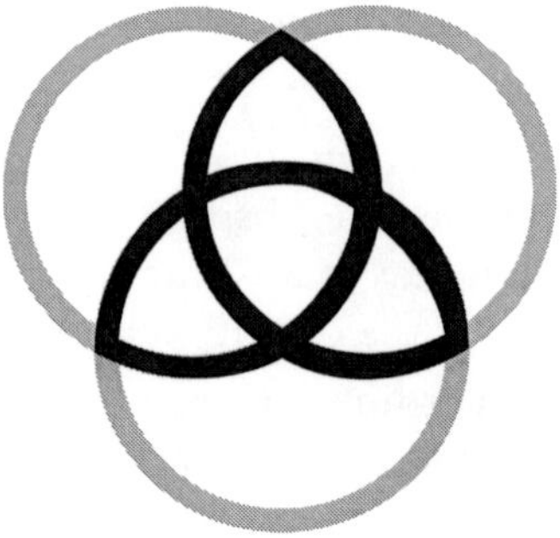

Draw this Figure: Draw a circle and draw a circle horizontally mid-way over it leaving space on both sides of the original circle. Draw the following figures.

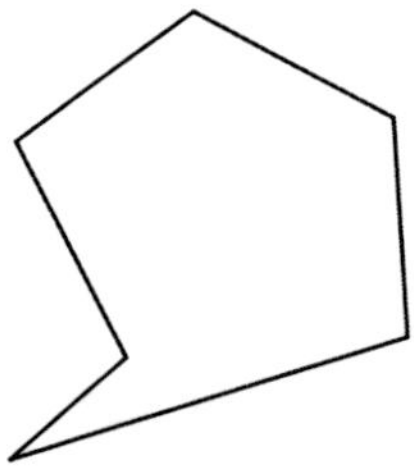

Irregular Hexagon

The drawings with angles help with sense of directions.

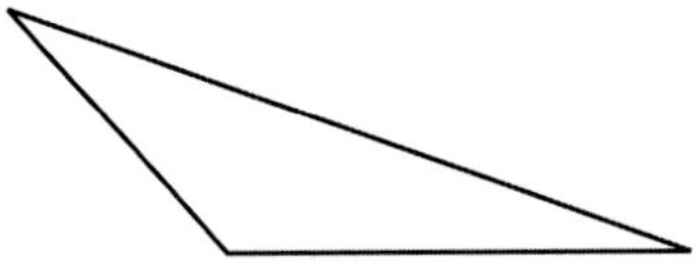

Obtuse Triangle

You can request ADIs to draw anything they like as long as they can say what they are and the meaning of these figures or drawings.

Generally, people like to draw a house, a person and a tree when asked to draw a picture. So much so there is a test called HTP (house, tree, person). When the ADI is asked to talk about HTP they drew, it may reveal many aspects of their lives. It may reveal several emotions as well. Give a bunch of colored pencils to draw and the colors that they use also will reveal the emotions. One can make them to talk of colors they like and that may reveal the types of dress they like to wear or even how their bedroom should be decorated.

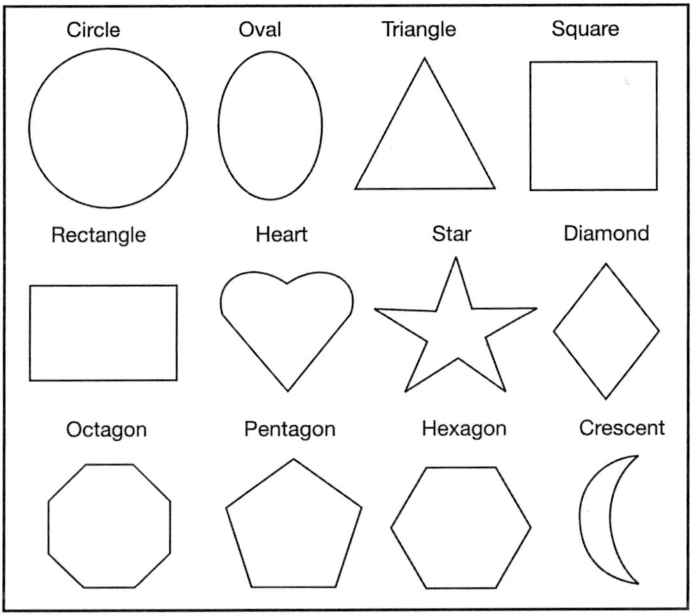

Draw these pictures to improve eye-hand coordination, visual perception, visual imagery and try to remember as many objects as you can. After drawing, name them. This inculcates a sense of direction as well and spatial relationships (Wikipedia Encyclopedia).

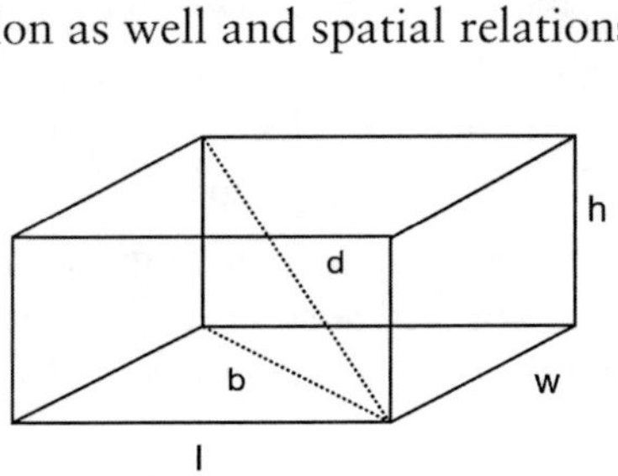

Source: Google

Drawing geometrical figures may help with directions, sense of locations to improve eye-hand coordination and stimulate parietal lobe.

Make clients to practice on Bender Gestalt type of figures. Simple to complex figures to improve parietal lobe functions as well as other lobes.

Bender Gestalt Test (Wikipedia has the picture of the test) was one time so famous that one of my professors had it printed on his tie. The first figure may look simple but for a patient it is difficult to make the angles and connect the diamond to the circle.

The following figures and drawings will help with eye-hand coordination perceptual and, motor proficiency, sense of balance, ability to analyze and synthesize, sense of direction and so on. The figures in the test may be improvised for the Alzheimer's to improve overall cognition and eye-hand coordination.

Figure 1. On dot counting and reproducing the figure, brain impaired people may miss several dots and the line may not be straight.

On figure 2 the dots may be translated into circles and the slants may be ignored and the correct number of dots may be missing. The circle can be enlarged or minimized.

Continued training in drawing will improve the eye-hand coordination and motor proficiency and visual perception.

The seventh figure poses insurmountable difficulty to brain impaired patients. The proportion and angulations are altered and may not recognize that the stimulus figure is altered beyond recognition. With practice the abilities required to perform the test will improve. Will give more confidence to the patient.

The 8th figure can be altered altogether by the brain impaired people. Do not diagnose brain impairment on the basis of any one test. If these figures are difficult for the ADIs, select drawings that are simple.

Games must be fun and interactive. The activities must give them a feeling of importance, autonomy, happiness and socially productive. Some of them may be able to write a skit and people can enact. Memories of childhood activities may be recalled. Cooking, menu planning, cooking and eating together may give them a sense of confidence in social situations and empowerment. This is also social engagement. Tests mentioned in this book can be improvised and practiced to improve cognitive abilities. The chapter on Neuropsychological Tests will be handy to improve all aspects of attention, language, thinking, learning, memory, executive functions, visual perception and so on to adapt to situations. Neuroscientists are working hard to improve the lot of Alzheimer's patients.

Each person seated in a circle, writes-in a few words, fold it to conceal part of the writing and pass it on to the next person to write down a few words. Do not stop. Continue to play. After about three trials read the completed paper. The result should tell the examiner the progress of the Alzheimer's language and communication abilities. Make each person to correct their thoughts if necessary. The variant to this is completing the drawing of a person. This can be fun and hilarious.

Hide a few things but letting the patient know where it is kept. After 10 minutes ask the patient to find them in the order they are kept.

Ask each one to tell a story. This will encourage the patient to talk. Others can help a patient by completing the thoughts if the person gets stuck. Make everyone to read a poem out loud. This helps reading, relieve stress and anxiety and get rid of stage fright.

It is recommended that people with memory disturbances play brain games till they are not able to play. Depending on which games one plays, this strengthens brain skills including memory, concentration, problem-solving, thinking speed, and mental flexibility. Options include hundreds of free games on the Internet. People can subscribe to brain games services like Luminosity. Cambridge Brain Sciences Inc. provides scientifically proven tools for the assessment of cognitive functions over the web. It is free. The test measures memory, reasoning, concentration and planning. There are many sites to play cognitive games.

What are the things the government can do for you? And what are things your government can learn from other countries?

What should your community do for you?

How will you change the health system to serve you?

Mild Alzheimer's may want to give a try on the following:

For memorization, use the memory systems such as the peg, journey; memory palace; name-face and phonetic number methods. These systems involve using the visualization memory technique.

Visual input creates the strongest recall value of all senses, and also allows the widest spectrum of levels-of-processing modifiers. Within visual studies, pictures have been shown to have a greater recall value than words—the picture superiority effect; followed by auditory stimuli. In other words, color has the potential to increase chances of environmental stimuli to be encoded, stored, and retrieved successfully. Auditory stimuli (spoken words and sounds) have the highest recall value when spoken, and visual stimuli have the highest recall value when a subject is presented with images. Tactile memory representations are similar in nature to visual representations, although there is not enough data to reliably compare the strength of the two kinds of stimuli.

Smell

Odor memory is weaker than visual memory, achieving a successful identification rate of only 70-80 per cent of visual memory (levels of processing effect from Wikipedia, the free encyclopedia).

For mental exercises, weave memory exercises into daily routine to strengthen memory. Mental snapshots are good to improve episodic memory of events, it takes a mental snapshot of important scenes and special moments. Researchers at Stanford University's Memory Laboratory showed that the more subjects forgot competing memories, the less work their brains had to do to recall a specific one. So a certain degree of forgetting is completely normal.

Cognitive Stimulation Therapy is an intervention for people with dementia that offers a range of enjoyable activities providing general stimulation for thinking, concentration and memory, usually in a social setting such as a small group. It is aimed at general enhancement of cognitive and social functioning. Family caregivers can be trained to provide cognitive stimulation on a one-to-one basis.

The use of group CST is growing rapidly in the UK and internationally, yet many people with dementia may be unable or unwilling to participate in group CST.

"Societal needs: (NICE) With increasing number of dementia anticipated in coming years, a group approach to CST intervention will allow for fiscal conservancy of insurance monies while providing an environment for best results of CST. CST recommends social interaction for the development of language skills and communication into CST protocols. This approach to dementia care will also provide a non-pharmacological alternative for chemical restraint reduction programs which are a current standard for medicare. On evaluation of its efficacy, the results clearly showed that those who were given the Cognitive Stimulation Therapy did significantly better on all memory tasks than those that did not receive the therapy. Some health insurance companies deny coverage for Cognitive Stimulation Therapy."

"Individual Cognitive Stimulation (iCST) is based on the evidence-based group CST therapy for people with mild to moderate dementia, which has been found to be beneficial for cognition and quality of life. The iCST program is delivered by a relative or close friend of the person with dementia for: > 30 Minutes, >3 times a week; > over 25 weeks. Each individual CST session consists of a themed activity (i.e. life story, discussion of current affairs, being creative) and is designed to be mentally stimulating. The potential benefits of iCST include improved well-being for people with dementia and their caregivers. It is of economic and social benefits such as reduced costs of care and delayed institutionalization. iCST can also be offered in combination with anti-dementia medication. iCST provides an option for those unsuitable for or unwilling to take medication. It is possible that iCST program could be used widely across in UK and internationally" (US National Library of Medicine, National Institutes of Health Journal List PMC 3522062).

ADIs and caregivers in England recognize the need for Individualized CST. Studies report that "home-based memory management program involving family caregivers lead to improvements in memory in the person with dementia. A few studies have focused on the use of cognitive stimulation programs in the home environment. In a pilot study, Moniz-Cook et al. found that a home-based memory management program involving the family caregiver led to improvements in memory in the person with dementia, improvements in caregiver well-being, and a reduction in care home admissions at 18 months".

Alzheimer's Disease: Tips for Maintaining a Normal Life at home

- To help cope with memory problems in case of advanced AD to a moderate level.
- Record in a book important information, phone numbers, names, ideas you have, appointments, your address, and directions to your home. Keep track of your movements. If you are going for a walk, remember important landmarks and note directions.
- Stick notes at a proper place in the house to remind self of activities and duties.
- Label cupboards and drawers in writing that describe their contents. Remove what you do not use. Do not clutter the cupboards.
- Place important phone numbers in large print next to the phone.
- Ask a friend or family member to call and remind you of important things that you need to do in the day, like meal times, medication times, and appointments. (In India generally ADIs live with the family and help the ADI with most of these things.)
- Use a calendar to be oriented to date and month and to remember important dates of events like birthdays of friends and relatives.

- Look through photos of people labeled with their names not to forget them.
- Keep track of phone messages in a phone notebook kept near the phone. In India not many homes have the luxury of possessing an answering machine. Many older people are reluctant to use a mobile phone even. Some of them can be taught to use the mobile phone.
- Put on very soothing and relaxing music through intercom.

Ultimate question is how to improve cognitive and executive functions. Activities of daily living (ADL) refers to self-care activities. Another domain, related to ADLs and IADLs (Instrumental ADL), is cognitive ability. Cognitive impairment and ADL status are correlated but are separate dimensions of functioning according to some psychologists. Not all persons with substantial cognitive impairment have ADL dysfunctions.

Mild to moderate ADIs are able to perform ADLs and IADLs with some assistance and guidance. They are good candidates to train on cognitive stimulation so that they can function in the community without much assistance.

Individual cognitive stimulation coordinated with caregivers will be far more effective than just group training. Individual program can be tailored according to their cognitive abilities.

Basic ADLs (BADLs) consist of self-care tasks, including:

Set a specific time to get up in the morning. Some people may be able to set the time on technical devices that are available like a clock, mobile phone and the like. Time to wake up can be behaviorally conditioned.

The ability to prepare a cup of tea/coffee. Ability to make it in a microwave or percolators. If a cook is employed, ADI must have the ability to ask for the morning coffee. Should have the ability to make that arrangement.

Attend to natures call without difficulties and wash up after. Some people do not know how to use a toilet faucet in India. Teach them how to use properly. In India this may be a problem because of lack of facilities. Most middle class has this facility. (Some people have difficulties using these facilities because of cultural interpretations of the practice being unhealthy.)

Personal Hygiene and Grooming: Allow the person to have a bath by self if that is possible but be attentive. Do not allow the person to be in the bathroom all by herself or himself because of fear of falling. Person should leave the bathroom door unlocked. ADI should be aware of dangers. Arrange all toiletries and cosmetics systematically so that the patient can reach them and without much effort physically and mentally. At times minor inconveniences can make them agitated. Patient should be taught about the temperature of bath water and after the bath, patient may be informed that the body may be wiped with a soft towel and must wipe all the folds.

To be dressed in appropriate attire is important to everyone. ADIs may have their preferences for the color and special attire. Train ADIs to select the appropriate dress, carry out grooming, putting on clothes, shoes and other activities that come under grooming. Personal grooming involves various aspects such as hair, skin, nails, teeth, and make up. ADI should be aware of self care.

ADI should be aware of proper eating/feeding (including chewing and swallowing). Inadequate food and fluid intake can result in malnutrition, dehydration, skin breakdown and other difficulties.

Functional mobility is moving from one place to another while performing activities. If the ADIs can function on the three mobility domains as walking, stance, and rising from chair, the ADIs may be able to do some chores. Walking may be the best predictor of overall functional mobility.

Train in daily activities so that the patient will maintain daily routines. This may reduce stress and confusion. Do the same thing, the same time so that biological clock is maintained.

Instrumental ADLs: Instrumental Activities of Daily Living (IADLs)

Housework and basic home maintenance: In India maids are available to do house work for those who can afford them. Middle class can afford cooks and maids. Most of them are reliable and some of them are live ins. ADIs should be able to supervise the work.

Administering own medications as prescribed. Most of them will be able to follow instructions and with the help of the container with days of the week mentioned.

Keep appointments with physicians and others and make arrangements to keep the appointments.

Managing money: In India, older people rely on other family members. If one can manage one's own funds, it will give more independence. In India, it is better to seek help from a trusted source.

Make a list for shopping for groceries or clothing. Shopping for clothes can be done with the help of another family member if need be. If ADI has basic knowledge of computers, the person should be able to order for groceries and clothing on line.

Use of telephone and other technical devices.

Use Transportation within the community instead of driving. In India, it will be difficult for older people to use public transportation. Can make arrangements with reliable auto rickshaw/cab owners. Beware some people can cheat the older folks.

Keep phone numbers of your neighbors, relatives and friends to get in touch with if need arises (if the person is living alone). It is rare that a middle class person will be living alone in India.

Both ADLs and IADLs skills are absolutely necessary to survive as independent individuals in any society. However, middle-class individuals have the luxury of help from family members and hired hands.

University of Nebraska medical center has a scale for instrumental activities of daily living to assess the following:

1. Ability to use telephone
2. Shopping
3. Food preparation
4. Housekeeping
5. Laundry
6. Mode of transportation
7. Responsibility for own medication
8. Ability to handle finances.

In India, most middle-class people, even low middle class can employ someone to help with these activities; even can hire someone 24/7.

"Most researchers are in agreement that cognitive training can help some of the people some of the time." Hard work at cognitive training improves cognitive functions.

Scientific American: Can cognitive training make you smarter? Interview with author Dan Hurley, science journalist, "what kind of effect does cognitive training have on the brain?"

"There is no question that training causes structural and functional improvement in the brain, as seen on MRI. Most of the changes are seen in the frontal areas of the brain, where high-level thinking occurs. Mindfulness meditation, for instance, has been shown to produce increased white-matter connections between the anterior cingulate cortex, an important region for complex decision-making, and the rest of the brain."

Alzheimer's Disease: Utilize Community Resources

Provide community-based physical activity programs that offer mild forms of aerobics and other exercises suitable to AD patients for strengthening muscles, and flexibility components specifically designed for older adults. ADIs must be informed about the advantages of these activities. In India, walking activities will be best to improve the health of the older people.

Encourage malls and other indoor or protected locations to provide safe places for walking in any weather. Indian

Government must advice builders of homes and apartments to use non-skid tiles so that older people or for that or for that matter no one should skid, fall and break bones skid, fall and break bones. It is the concern of many older people, I talked to regarding flight of stairs in office buildings like banks and post offices.

There are well-planned parks in Chennai and Bungaluru. Park authorities may want to involve the older people in the design of Parks and gardens. Nature can be brought to parks and gardens for the enjoyment of the older people. Design special parks only for older people and with proper security. Have programs for ADIs and families on TVs with the intention to entertain and educate.

Ensure that facilities for physical activity accommodate and encourage participation by older adults. India has to make an assessment of such facilities to find out whether these facilities are adequate, safe and cater to the needs of the elderly and ADIs. Most elderly spend their time at home not knowing what is available in the community for activities.

Provide transportation for older adults to parks or facilities that provide physical activity programs for elderly.

Encourage health care providers to talk routinely to their older adult patients about incorporating physical activity into their lives (This is rare in India). However, Yoga is available.

Plan community activities that include opportunities for older adults to be physically active. Use school premises for activities. In USA, people use school auditorium, its swimming pool and other facilities for community activities. Seniors use shopping malls for early morning walks. Community Mental Health facilities in USA provide such facilities.

Indian government has to allot money in several crores to set up programs for Alzheimer's and generally for elderly.

"It is important that people with dementia are treated with respect and their dignity is maintained. It is also important to remember that a person with dementia is still a unique and valuable being, despite illness" (Alzheimer's Society).

REFERENCES

Aging & Mental Health (1998). 2:199-211. PubMed Abstract

Glisky & GliskyGlisky, E.L. & Glisky, M.L. (1999). Memory rehabilitation in theelderly. In D.T. Stuss, G. Winocur, & I.H. Robertson (Eds.) Cognitive rehabilitation (pp. 347-61). Cambridge: Cambridge University Press.

Moniz-Cook E., Agar S., Gibson G., Win T., Wang M. A preliminary study of the effects of early intervention with people with dementia and their families in a memory clinic.

Wilson, Barnes, and Bennett, 2003; Wilson et al. (2002) Wilson, R., Barnes, L., & Bennett, D. (2003). Assessment of lifetime participation in cognitively stimulating activities. *Journal of Clinical and Experimental Neuropsychology*, 25(5), 634-42.

Wilson, R.S., Mendes De Leon, C.F., Barnes, L.L., Schneider, J.A., Biennia's, J.L., Evans, D.A., & Bennett, D.A. (2002). Participation in cognitively stimulating activities and risk of incident Alzheimer disease. *The Journal of the American Medical Association*, 287(6), 742-48.

Yaffe, K., Barnes, D., Nevitt, M., Lui, L.Y., & Covinsky, K. (2001). A prospective study of physical activity and cognitive decline in elderly Yaffe, K., Barnes, D., Nevitt, M., Lui, L.Y., & Covinsky, K. (2001). A prospective study of physical activity and cognitive decline in elderly women: Women who walk. *Archives of Internal Medicine*, 161(14), 1703-708.